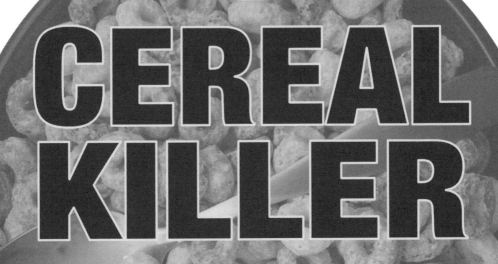

CEREAL KILLER

The Unintended Consequences of the Low Fat Diet

By ALAN L. WATSON

Published by **Diet Heart Publishing**

DISCLAIMER: The information in this book is for educational purposes only. Neither the publisher nor the author is engaged in rendering professional advice or services to the individual reader. All matters regarding physical health should be supervised by a health practitioner knowledgeable in treating your particular condition. Neither the author nor the publisher shall be liable or responsible for any loss, injury, or damage allegedly arising from any information or suggestion in this book.

CEREAL KILLER

Copyright © 2008, Alan L. Watson
3rd Printing — February 2010

ISBN 978-0-9720481-1-8

Published by Diet Heart Publishing
2235 E 38th St., Minneapolis, MN 55407

You can reach the publisher on the internet at www.dietheartpublishing.com.

Graphic design by Jezac Design: www.jezac.com
Cover Photo by Jesse Thomas, Minneapolis, MN

Printed in the United States of America

❧ *Acknowledgements* ❧

I am indebted to scores of medical doctors and researchers whose published results and clinical data form the scientific basis of this book.

A particular note of gratitude goes to the late Weston A. Price and the late Dr. Robert C. Atkins — *American heroes* — pioneers in the critically important effort to restore America's high fat, whole foods daily fare.

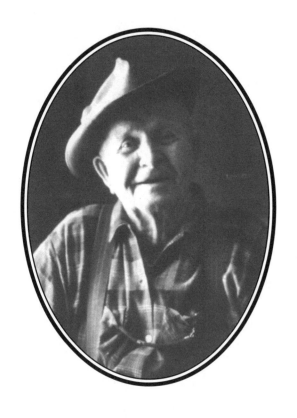

*Dedicated to the memory of my
grandfather Robert T. Komula, a pioneer
Minnesota dairy farmer who knew how to farm,
what to eat for breakfast – and after compulsory
nationwide pasteurization in 1949,
knew it was time to quit.*

❧ *Table of Contents* ❧

Part I: The test of time **7**

    Chapter 1: Pyramid Schemes **11**

    Chapter 2: Lessons of Framingham **21**

    Chapter 3: Unintended Consequences **27**

    Chapter 4: Cereal Killer **35**

    Chapter 5: Class of 2018 . . . . **43**

Part II: Life in the fat lane **55**

    Chapter 6: 'Loose Lips Sink Ships' **59**

    Chapter 7: Atkins…without Atkins **67**

    Chapter 8: Cholesterol is not a Medical Criminal! . . **77**

    Chapter 9: Lipids for Smart People **85**

    Chapter 10: Praise the Lard **99**

Epilogue: Be careful with whom you trust your heart **109**

Notes **113**

Appendix 1: Lipid Panel — Summary of coronary
                heart disease risk factors **120**

Appendix 2: Lipids — The Big Picture **123**

Index **138**

FALLUJA, Iraq, Nov 23 (*Reuters*)

"Braving snipers, Falluja residents walked past demolished homes to an aid distribution centre on Tuesday but American granola bars and Frosted Flakes cereal failed to raise hopes of a brighter future…"

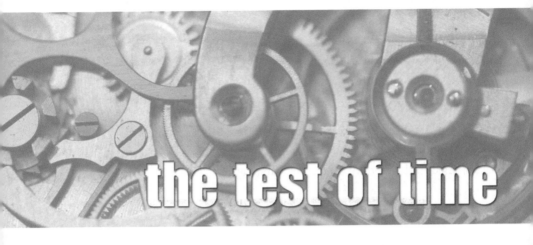

the test of time

"The age is ending, the house is coming down
– all the rafters, all the towers, all the clocks.
It was built of a dream. The dream closes."

— *Allen Wheelis*

SUMMER, 2008.

A record number of American children are being diagnosed with asthma, obesity, Type 2 diabetes, and bipolar disorder. Along with surging food and medical costs, Americans must come to grips with declining life expectancy — now 37th in the world.

According to the Center for Disease Control in Atlanta, the number of American children who became overweight tripled during the 1980s. Type 2 diabetes followed apace.

Today, 65 percent of all Americans are overweight or obese — more than 25 million are diabetic.

Health insurance premiums are climbing too as trillions are spent for disease management — not cures. Aghast at the number of Americans without health insurance, well meaning politicians are calling for universal health care, even though, after decades of food warring, our medical and scientific communities can't even agree on what constitutes a healthy breakfast.

The "low fat diet," first promoted by the nonprofit American Heart Association in 1961, came with the promise to end heart disease:

> "If everyone were to [lower their fat intake], coronary bypass surgery would be rare by the end of the century."[1]

In 1977, the federal government adopted the American Heart Association's "low fat" diet. We reduced fat, increased grains and cereal, and switched to the recommended vegetable fats.

> Bacon, butter, chicken skin, coconut oil, egg yolk, creamy lard, and red meat were fingered as the cause of everything!

Unrelenting media attacked traditional foods. The soybean-oil-friendly Center for Science in the Public Interest (CSPI) launched their "Anti-Saturated Fat Attack" against coconut oil and butter in movie theatre popcorn. Replaced by

> — you guessed it — partially hydrogenated soybean oil and imitation butter.

In 1987, the medical elite announced their long-awaited "War on Cholesterol," launching what has become the Titanic of needless medical interventions. In his book *Heart Failure*, Thomas J. Moore describes it this way:

> "Like some ponderous prehistoric beast, the National Cholesterol Education Program just slowly surfaced from the bureaucratic swamps at the heart institute."[3]

By decree, 25 million Americans were battling a new enemy — *high cholesterol*. That same year, Merck's Lovastatin, the first cholesterol-lowering statin drug, was approved in record time — 12 weeks.

Dr. Scott Grundy, American Heart Association board member and paid consultant to Merck, wrote a favorable nine-page article about Lovastatin in the *New England Journal of Medicine*. Doctor-consultants like Grundy helped make the "War on Cholesterol" a big success.

But, instead of victory, heart disease remains the number one killer, and slow, suffocating heart failure is the number one Medicare expenditure. And, as an example, since the year 2000, five new specialty heart hospitals have opened just in the Minneapolis and St. Paul metro area.[2]

The decades-old War on Cholesterol became a great, everlasting marketing opportunity for the giant U.S. cereal businesses — all founding members of the National Cholesterol Education Program.

> For a fee, *high glycemic* breakfast bars, sugary Pop Tarts,®
> and Yogurt Burst Cheerios® could earn the American Heart
> Association's *low fat* seal of approval.

Now, in a time of war, is it unpatriotic to ask whether the medical and business elite have let us down and put their personal and financial interests ahead of everything else, like our health?

Very possible, says award-winning science writer Gary Taubes, author of *Good Calories, Bad Calories*. The curtain is falling on "low fat," says Taubes, and what we have now is the test of time…

> "And, the idea that eating less fat makes for a healthier and
> longer life has only become less compelling over time."[4]

Cereal Killer is a history of the low fat era. Dry boxed cereal is a metaphor for all that's gone wrong with our food supply. As Americans suffer from a balkanized scientific establishment, the big cereal and pharmaceutical industries enjoy record profits.

But the chickens will come home to roost, and the *unintended consequences* are filling up the hen house.

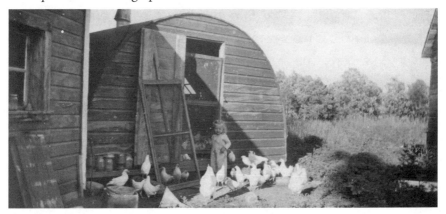

Follow the money...

Expect a Food Fight As U.S. Revises Dietary Guidelines

As reported in the August 8, 2003, *Wall Street Journal*, "After months of behind-the-scenes jockeying by commodity groups and nutrition advocates, the federal government is expected to announce as early as today which scientists and other experts will revise the nation's dietary guidelines."[5]

According to the story, "the Sugar Association and Soft Drink Association were jockeying behind the scenes."[6] These industry lobbyists and nutritionists, no doubt, will fight hard to ensure that the "Class of 2018" gets at least 10 teaspoons or more of sugar in each soft drink, breakfast pastry, or serving of boxed cereal.

During the 2000 revision (the guidelines are revised every five years), Sean McBride, a spokesman for the Soft Drink Association, was pleased with his success in watering down any warnings about the danger of dietary sugar:

"We plan to work with the panel again [in 2005] to counter allegations from the activist community, and public misperceptions that there is evidence to link sugar and obesity," he says.[7]

According to the *Wall Street Journal*, the 13-member panel that revises the federal nutrition guidelines "must include nutrition experts who are leaders in the fields of pediatrics, obesity, cardiovascular disease and public health...."[8]

"Industry groups know the opinions of many of the experts, at least partly because many nutrition researchers are affiliated with them, serving on their boards, doing research and taking on speaking engagements."[9]

CHAPTER 1

Pyramid Schemes

"In America, we no longer fear God or the communists, but we fear fat."
— *David Kritchevsky, Wistar Institute*

Until the early 1950s, eggs, butter, cream, lard, and red meat from pastured animals were considered nutritious foods. Small, mixed family farms and busy creameries dotted the landscape. Dairy was the largest employer, producing and distributing abundant raw milk and products made from raw milk.

Family Fare, Home and Garden Bulletin No. 1, February 1950, U.S. Department of Agriculture (USDA), had this to say about complete protein:

> "The best quality proteins have all of the important amino acids and worthwhile amounts of each. You get top-rating proteins in foods from animal sources, as in meat, poultry, fish, eggs, milk and cheese."[1]

The current 2005 federal nutrition guidelines don't say one word about "complete protein," nor do they mention the importance of fat soluble vitamins A and D. *Family Fare* emphasized eating wholesome foods that provide plenty of vitamin A:

> "You can get vitamin A from animal foods. Good sources

are liver, egg yolks, butter, whole milk and cream, and cheese made from whole milk or cream. Fish liver oils which children take for vitamin D are rich in vitamin A besides…"[2]

Then, beginning in the 1950s, foods eaten for generations were fingered by the American Heart Association as the cause of heart disease. Reported deaths from coronary heart disease were rising, and a reorganized, fundraising American Heart Association blamed the increase on cholesterol and saturated fat.

In 1953, Ancel Keys, American Heart Association board member and professor at the University of Minnesota, published his *Six Countries Analysis*, showing a correlation between dietary fat and heart disease in six of 22 countries. By ignoring data from 16 countries, Keys was able to argue that fat *caused* heart disease.

But association or correlation is not causation! As an example, the U.S. had a relatively high fat diet and high rates of heart disease. The Japanese had a very low fat diet and low rates of heart disease. But, after the war, the Japanese also had very low calorie diets, low consumption of sugar and refined foods, and a much higher rate of deadly strokes — associations Keys ignored.

"Low fat" began on television in 1956 when American Heart Association doctors conducting a fundraiser told a national TV audience to replace traditional American foods — eggs, butter and red meat — with boxed cereal, margarine, vegetable shortening, polyunsaturated corn oil and skinless chicken.

Five years later, AHA board member Ancel Keys was famous. He had made the cover of *Time* (January 13, 1961), and at his urging, the American Heart Association officially adopted his "low fat" high carbohydrate diet. Fellow board member and University of Chicago professor Jeremiah Stamler was a staunch Keys backer.

Stamler was the author of *Your Heart Has Nine Lives*, a self-help book advocating the substitution of vegetable oils for butter and other so-called "artery clogging saturated fats." The book and Stamler's research were sponsored by the makers of Mazola Corn Oil and Fleischmann's Margarine. Stamler said it was time to recommend low fat — and vegetable fat —

"even before the final proof is nailed down."[3]

Over time, the American Heart Association's anti-fat position became increasingly rigid. By 1970, "low fat" applied not only to high risk men who had high cholesterol or smoked but to everyone over age 2, including:

> "infants, children, adolescents, pregnant and lactating women, and older persons."

Published in 1970, Keys' *Seven Countries Study* only fueled the scientific controversy. According to *Good Calories, Bad Calories* author Gary Taubes, "Keys chose seven countries he knew in advance would support his anti-fat hypothesis." As an example, Keys ignored Switzerland and France, countries with high animal fat diets and low rates of heart disease (true today).[4]

In 1977, Senator George McGovern settled politically what could not be settled scientifically. This was post Viet Nam 1977 when big American appetites came under scrutiny. After two series of contentious hearings, McGovern's extra-legislative bipartisan Committee on Nutrition and Human Needs adopted *defacto* the AHA "low fat" diet.

According to Taubes, McGovern's young, idealistic staff of lawyers and ex-journalists had no scientific training. Nick Mottern, a vegetarian and former labor reporter for a Rhode Island newspaper, "almost single-handedly" drafted the committee's *Dietary Goals for the United States*.[5]

For the first time, a branch of the federal government told the American public that eating more carbohydrates and less fat was healthy. A client of the Pritikin low fat program, a pudgy Senator McGovern went into the hearings biased in favor of the American Heart Association's low fat, high carbohydrate diet.

According to Taubes:

> "*Dietary Goals* sparked a chain reaction of dietary advice from government agencies and the press that reverberate still, and the document itself became gospel."[6]

Since then, it's been a green light for carbohydrates –flashing red for fat. Between 1980 and 2005, federal nutrition guidelines have recommended that up to 65 percent of our daily calories come from carbohydrates. The 2005 revised guidelines say:

> "Choose fiber-rich fruits, vegetables, and whole grains

often. Choosing plenty of these foods, within the context
of a calorie-controlled diet, can promote health and reduce
chronic disease."[7]

Fingered by the American Heart Association as the cause of heart
disease, dietary fat, especially saturated fat and cholesterol, was to be eaten
sparingly. Choose "lean, low fat or fat free." Since 1980, the guidelines have
contained the American Heart Association's fear-based, anti-fat directive:

> Consume *less than* 30 percent of calories as fat, *less than* 10
> percent of calories as saturated fat, and *less than* 300 mg of
> cholesterol daily.[8]

In 1987, an alliance of doctors from the American Heart Association
and the National Institutes of Health, joined by a public relations armada
of food, medical and pharmaceutical companies, launched the *National
Cholesterol Education Program*, the long-awaited war against cholesterol.

Cholesterol reduction became the single focus of heart disease research and treatment. "Exercise and eat a low-fat diet," they say, and if that
doesn't lower your cholesterol enough, "take a drug for the rest of your life."
This is the American Heart Association hypothesis, also referred to as the
cholesterol or lipid theory of heart disease.

The American Heart Association's low fat mantra was now being
amplified by the U.S. Department of Agriculture, the National Institutes
of Health, dietitians, health organizations, consumer groups, reporters,
cookbook writers and book publishers.

Throughout McGraw-Hill's textbook, *Perspectives in Nutrition* (1999),
there are warnings linking saturated fat to the various "killer diseases."
Students are repeatedly instructed to reduce saturated fat in their diets:

> "To reduce saturated fat, use tub margarine instead of but-
> ter... Season vegetables with herbs and spices rather than
> with sauces or butter...Use applesauce and other fruit purees
> in place of fat...Replace whole milk with nonfat milk...Limit
> bacon, ribs, and meatloaf... Remove skin from poultry before
> cooking...Limit high fat cheese..."[9]

When you reduce fat, you must increase something. Grain
consumption increased 60 pounds per capita since 1980; high fructose
corn syrup 30 pounds. Today, nearly 10 percent of the calories Americans

consume come from corn sweeteners. (For children the figure is 20 percent.)

In response to the National Cholesterol Education Program, Russell Smith, Ph.D., statistician and author of two scientific papers critical of the lipid hypothesis, said:

> "The current campaign to convince every American to change his or her diet, and in many cases, to initiate drug therapy for life is based on fabrications, erroneous interpretations, and/or gross exaggerations of findings and, very importantly, the ignoring of massive amounts of unsupportive data."[10]

During the "low fat" era, obesity, which had remained constant from the early 1960s through 1980, developed into a major public health issue. Because obesity and diabetes increase heart disease risk, the incidence of heart disease has not gone down as promised. And heart failure — a suffocating enlargement of the heart — has become the number one Medicare expenditure.

Alice and Fred Ottoboni, researchers with PhD's respectively in Comparative Biochemistry and Environmental Health Sciences, blame obesity, diabetes, and heart disease on the federal nutrition guidelines and Americans' increased consumption of sugar, grain, and vegetable fat — especially trans fat:

> "The USDA-sponsored Dietary Guidelines for Americans and its Food Guide Pyramid are nutritionally and biochemically unsound. The Dietary Guidelines for Americans was nevertheless accepted wholeheartedly by nutrition authorities who took Ancel Keys as their guiding spirit and his lipid hypothesis as their mantra."[11]

In their excellent book, *The Modern Nutritional Diseases*, the Ottoboni's document how the last hundred years have seen widespread dietary changes that are incompatible with human biochemical processes. They write:

> "Humans are not genetically programmed to be healthy on diets that are rich in omega-6 fatty acids [vegetable fat], sugar, starch, and trans fats…."[11]

The Ottoboni's write, "the Food Guide Pyramid has radically changed the food habits of tens of millions of Americans in a massive human experiment that has gone awry." The assertion in the guidelines that saturated fat causes heart disease has led to a fear of fat that:

> "Prevents a reasonable and balanced intake of dietary lipids and leads to a critical deficiency of saturated fats, an unnecessary limitation on cholesterol, and an unhealthful ratio of omega 6 and omega 3 essential fatty acids."[12]

The latest incarnation of the Food Guide Pyramid, released in April 2005, encourages us to replace some of the refined grains we've been eating with whole grains. While the emphasis on whole grains is new, the 2005 revision adheres to the cholesterol- and fat-phobic diet the AHA began promoting in 1961.

Well conducted, long term studies "T-bone" the lipid hypothesis. In the Nurses' Health Studies (I and II) and in the Health Professionals Follow-Up Study, the Harvard School of Public Health accumulated data on the diet and health of over 300,000 Americans. Those data, says Harvard's Walter Willet:

> "Clearly contradict the low-fat-is-good-health message."[13]

The results suggest that "total fat consumed has no relation to heart disease risk" and "nurses who ate less fat seemed to have more breast cancer."[14, 15] In an interview with Taubes, Willett, spokesperson for the Nurses' Health Study, pointed out that the federal government spent over $100 million on the Harvard studies and yet not one government agency has changed its guidelines to fit the data. "Scandalous," said Willet.

> "They say you really need a high level of proof to change the recommendations, which is ironic, because they never had a high level of proof to set them."[16]

"The USDA food pyramid nutrition recommendations are dead wrong."

— *William Campbell Douglass, M.D.*

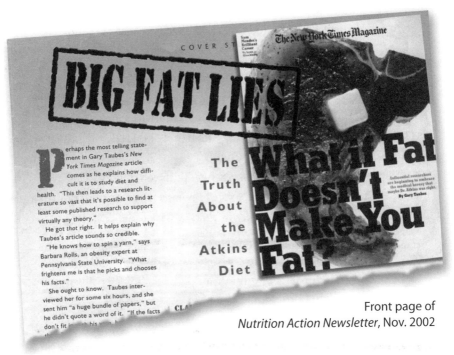

Perhaps the most telling statement in Gary Taubes's *New York Times Magazine* article comes as he explains how difficult it is to study diet and health. "This then leads to a research literature so vast that it's possible to find at least some published research to support virtually any theory."

He got *that* right. It helps explain why Taubes's article sounds so credible.

"He knows how to spin a yarn," says Barbara Rolls, an obesity expert at Pennsylvania State University. "What frightens me is that he picks and chooses his facts."

She ought to know. Taubes interviewed her for some six hours, and she sent him "a huge bundle of papers," but he didn't quote a word of it. "If the facts don't fit in...his...

The Truth About the Atkins Diet

Front page of
Nutrition Action Newsletter, Nov. 2002

BIG **FAT** LIES

In response to Gary Taubes' front page *NY Times Magazine* article, "What if Fat Doesn't Make You Fat," Michael Jacobson, the director of the 1980s *Anti-Saturated Fat Attack*, published a rebuttal cover story in his *Nutrition Action Newsletter* called "BIG FAT LIES, The Truth about the Atkins Diet."

Several of the medical researchers Taubes had interviewed were forced to reaffirm the American Heart Association party line.

> "Gary Taubes tricked us all into coming across as supporters of the Atkins diet," says John Farquhar, Stanford University.

> "It's preposterous. There's no real evidence that low-fat diets have caused the obesity epidemic," says Samuel Klein, Washington University School of Medicine.

> "It's silly to say that carbohydrates cause obesity. We're overweight because we overeat calories," says George Blackburn, Harvard University.

"My quote was correct, but the context suggested that I support eating saturated fat. I was horrified," says Gerald Reaven, Stanford University

Why would a knowledgeable medical scientist "be horrified" to support eating saturated fat? In the South Pacific and elsewhere, highly saturated coconut fat is associated with freedom from cancer and heart disease. Closer to home, *stearic acid* is the beneficial HDL-raising saturated fat found in chocolate, beef, and butter.

The consummate medical researcher, Taubes had good reason to interview Dr. Reaven, a respected expert on carbohydrate metabolism and the author of *Syndrome X, The Silent Killer*, in which he wrote:

> "Unknown millions of heart attacks have been caused by the failure of insulin, the body's "sugar cop," to do its job. This means that, for tens of millions of people, cholesterol is not the underlying problem leading to heart disease."[17]

On the back cover, the text reads, "If you have Syndrome X — and 60 to 75 million American do — the widely recommended low-fat, high carbohydrate diet may be the surest route to a heart attack."

No wonder Reaven found himself in the hot seat! Isn't this exactly what Dr. Atkins had been saying since 1972? (And what Gary Taubes concluded in *Good Calories, Bad Calories* after five years of full time research.)

If Reaven and other publicly funded researchers cast doubt on the prevailing nutritional wisdom, they could lose their funding. But if they defend a failed policy with forked tongues, they could be held accountable later on for ignoring the surging human and financial costs of obesity and diabetes.

Will the new, revised 2010 federal guidelines continue recommending excess grains and highly processed vegetable fats? What will convince the National Cholesterol Education Program to vote itself out of business? Will pyramid schemes and business lobbyists keep us on this road to ruin?

More to Explore...

One of the most important books on diet and health since the publication of Dr. Atkins Diet Revolution in 1972:

• Gary Taubes, *Good Calories, Bad Calories*, (New York: Alfred A. Knopf, 2007), published as *The Diet Delusion* in Great Britain in 2008 by Vermilion.

> The definitive book exploring all aspects of our failed nutrition guidelines. *Good Calories, Bad Calories* challenges the conventional wisdom on diet, weight control, and disease and makes a devastating case against the low-fat, high-carbohydrate way of life endorsed by the American Heart Association since 1961.

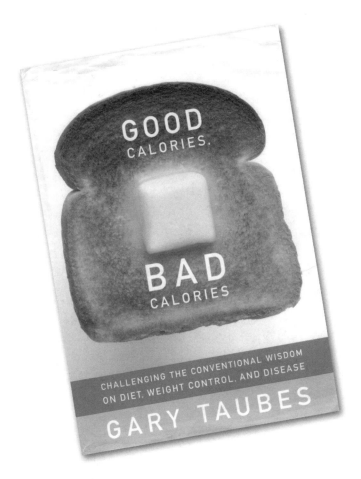

Oleomargarine May Be Dangerous

The editor of the *Jersey Bulletin* calls attention to recent experiments at the University of Minnesota under the direction of Dr. T.W. Gullickson on the relative merits of butterfat and oleo, and says: "Dr. Gullickson's experiments have confirmed what a lot of us have thought for a long time, that dairy calves fed whole milk thrive better than calves fed on skim milk with vegetable fats added in place of butterfat."

Experiments found that dairy calves fed vegetable fats in their diet invariably died by the time they were three months old. Some who were switched to a butterfat diet before three months survived. What these studies reveal is that calves fed corn oil to replace butterfat appear to show a vitamin E deficiency as indicated by heart lesions and muscle dystrophy or wasting of muscle tissue. This condition arises in spite of the high level of vitamin E in corn oil and is not corrected by adding vitamin E to the diet. More than 100 dairy calves have been used in these experiments.

"Reading reports of studies such as these leads us to wonder if part of the many, many persons who are dying of heart failure or attack each year that we have come to note in recent years could be attributed to our great switch to the use of oleomargarine in place of butter on the table. I am strongly convinced that it is some little thing such as the use of the 'yellowed imitation' that is taking its silent toll of human lives at too early an age."

— Sebeka Minnesota *Review* newspaper, March 11, 1953

CHAPTER 2

Lessons of Framingham

"In Framingham, Massachusetts, we found that the people who ate the most cholesterol, ate the most saturated fat, and ate the most calories, weighed the least and were the most physically active."
— *Dr. William P. Castelli, Director, Framingham Study, 1992*

In 1948, a team of Boston University Medical School researchers, sponsored by the National Institutes of Health, went to Framingham, Massachusetts to learn as much as possible about coronary heart disease — being reported in the U.S. at the time as the leading cause of death.

Framingham was primarily ethnic Irish and Italian, a blue-collar town of 28,000 people. The Boston University researchers wanted to learn who gets coronary heart disease — and what made them different from those who didn't. According to Thomas Moore's account in *Heart Failure,* 5,127 Framingham residents between the ages of 30 and 62 volunteered for the study.[1]

(The Framingham Study is epidemiology, the science that deals with the incidence, distribution, and control of a disease in a population.)

In no other city in the U.S. were a population's blood pressure, cholesterol levels, weight, and diet and exercise habits more systematically monitored. For decades, these Framingham residents would undergo physical exams, fill out detailed diet and lifestyle questionnaires, and be tested on exercise treadmills and electrocardiographs.

Framingham provided the now familiar heart disease *risk factors*: Advancing age, cigarette smoking, high blood pressure, obesity, and a sedentary lifestyle. And, men were much more likely to get heart disease than women, especially before age 55 (pre-menopausal women were practically immune).[2]

> Study participants with a combination of risk factors; i.e., older obese men who smoked and didn't exercise were much more likely to develop heart disease than non-smoking, trim younger men who walked a mile or two everyday.

Again, statistical association is not causation. Warnings were sounded when coffee drinking was positively associated with heart disease. When it was discovered that coffee drinkers were also more likely to smoke cigarettes — and cigarettes were the problem — the premature warning about coffee was withdrawn.

One early association drew special attention. Men between the ages of 30 and 48 who had higher than normal blood cholesterol were more likely to die of heart attacks.[3] But these middle-aged vulnerable men were also more likely to smoke, be overweight, or had familial hypercholesterolemia, a rare genetic condition that inactivates cholesterol receptors, causing very high levels of blood cholesterol to build up.[4]

This positive association between elevated cholesterol and heart disease in men under age 48 disappeared entirely once men reached 50. Since 90 percent of all heart attacks at that time occurred in people over 50, Framingham proved that:

> Blood cholesterol levels are not a risk factor for the majority of people who die of heart disease.[5]

Framingham also provided evidence that dietary cholesterol and saturated fat do not raise blood cholesterol or predispose a person to heart disease. Issued in 1970, "Diet and the Regulation of Serum Cholesterol" was a study of 912 Framingham residents that compared the cholesterol and fat in their diets with the cholesterol in their blood.

The researchers could find no relationship between dietary cholesterol and blood cholesterol; nor was there any relationship between saturated fat or calorie intake and blood cholesterol levels or risk of heart attack.

"There is a considerable range of serum cholesterol levels within the Framingham Study Group. Something explains this inter-individual variation, but it is not diet (as measured here)."[6]

In Framingham at the 20-year point (1971), there was extensive heart disease among study participants with low or borderline cholesterol (22 percent) and extensive heart disease among those with the highest cholesterol (18 percent).[7]

Average Serum Total Cholesterol	Occurrence of CHD
Low/Borderline TC (below 239)	22%
High TC (240 and above)	18%

(Average of 10 measurements over 20 years)

Since both low and high cholesterol can't cause heart disease, Framingham taught us that something other than cholesterol is causing heart disease. According to Thomas Yannios, M.D., "Framingham proved there is an 80 percent overlap of total cholesterol levels of those who do and do not get heart disease." In *Heart Disease Breakthrough*, Yannios wrote:

"In fact, many more people have heart disease and die of heart attacks at the lowest levels of cholesterol."[8]

At 30 years, the most dramatic finding in the Farmingham Study: Participants whose cholesterol levels had *declined* over the first 14 years ran a greater risk of dying from all causes than those whose cholesterol had *increased* over time.

"For each 1 mg/dl drop of cholesterol, there was an 11 percent increase in coronary and total mortality."[9]

That's worth repeating: Declining cholesterol was the best predictor of dying sooner! Never refuted, this finding raises a new question. If aging-related declining cholesterol is associated with earlier death, can deliberate cholesterol reduction with statin drugs shorten lives?

Yes, according to a study published in the *Journal of the American Geriatric Society*:

"Declining total cholesterol values in nursing home residents — losses greater than 45 mg/dl per year — increased the odds of mortality by more than six times."[10]

Blockbuster drugs like Lipitor are used by 25 million people worldwide, but a lot of research suggests their benefits are being oversold. According to *Business Week*, "Data suggest that for patients without heart disease, only 1 in 100 is likely to benefit from taking statin drugs."[11]

Medical doctor James M. Wright, a professor at the University of British Columbia, analyzed the evidence from years of statin drug trials. According to *Business Week*:

> "He found no benefit in people over the age of 65, no matter how much their cholesterol declines, and no benefit in woman of any age."[12]

"Most people are taking something with no chance of benefit and a risk of harm," says Dr Wright. In spite of this, the National Cholesterol Education Program says over 40 million of us — including very young children — should be taking cholesterol-lowering drugs.

Drug ads say you can reduce your risk of a heart attack by 36 percent if you take Lipitor.* But the truth is found in the small print they hope you don't read:

*"That means in a large clinical study, 3% of patients taking a sugar pill or placebo had a heart attack compared to 2% taking Lipitor."

Translated in print you can read: "For every 100 people in the trial, which lasted 3½ years, three people taking placebos and two people on Lipitor had heart attacks. The difference credited to the drug: One fewer heart attack per 100 people."[13] According to Dr. Wright:

> "To spare one person a heart attack, 100 people had to take Lipitor for more than three years. The other 99 got no measurable benefit."

Besides, higher blood cholesterol is protective in adults over 50. Low serum cholesterol is associated with death from accidents, cancer, and suicide. In a study of 7,603 male government employees, French researchers found that "the incidence of cancer began to climb steadily as cholesterol values fell below 200 mg/dl," the supposedly desirable level.[14]

Framingham, Dr. Wright's recent *Business Week* analysis, and dozens of other studies from around the world should have put an end to the unproven notion that saturated fat and dietary cholesterol increase blood cholesterol levels and cause heart disease. But like all findings that contradict the American Heart Association lipid hypothesis, they are simply ignored.

The Lessons of Framingham

- ❦ LDL and total cholesterol have little predictive significance for heart disease once people reach age 50.
- ❦ Dietary cholesterol doesn't increase blood cholesterol; nor does it increase the risk of heart disease.
- ❦ The majority of people who die of heart disease have low or average blood cholesterol.
- ❦ There was no relationship between sudden cardiac death and blood cholesterol levels after 24 years.
- ❦ Declining cholesterol over time was the best predictor of dying sooner of any cause.
- ❦ Something other than cholesterol and saturated fat are causing heart disease.

More to Explore...

The first great critical history of the failed "War on Cholesterol."

• Thomas J. Moore, *Heart Failure* (New York: Random House, 1989)

"A critical inquiry into why the public is being misled about the purported dangers of cholesterol. Heart Failure concludes that it was irresponsible to force the public into a costly cholesterol-reducing campaign without firm scientific evidence of its safety and effectiveness."

Patients with the highest cholesterol lived the longest!

In a study of 1,134 patients with advanced heart failure, low total cholesterol "was a strong, independent predictor of increased mortality." Low cholesterol was associated with "characteristics known to predict worse outcomes in heart failure," including decreased left ventricular ejection fraction — a key marker of heart failure.

Less than 25 percent of patients with total cholesterol in the lowest quintile (<129 mg/dl) survived five years, whereas survival was greater than 50 percent for patients in the two highest quintiles (>190 mg/dl).

The conclusion of the researchers:

> "This study clearly established that lower levels of total cholesterol and lipoproteins were associated with impaired survival in patients with heart failure, confirming the findings of the smaller, shorter-term studies."

Journal of the American College of Cardiology
Vol. 42, No. 11, 2003

CHAPTER 3

Unintended Consequences

"All reformers would do well to be conscious of the law of unintended consequences…"
— *Alan Stone, staff director, McGovern's Senate Committee*

In 1984, the president of the American Heart Association told *Time* magazine: "If everyone reduced their fat intake, we will have atherosclerosis conquered by the year 2000." Americans complied, consuming much more grain and grain products. We reduced our fat intake and continued our switch to the recommended vegetable fats.

So what's going on today? The American Heart Association is still raising millions of dollars (they have over $1 billion in assets); and throughout the world where populations have followed their dietary advice, the incidence of obesity and diabetes has increased at an alarming rate.

Is it possible that diabetes and obesity — *diabesity* as Atkins called it — share a single unifying cause and it's not the usual suspects, cholesterol and saturated fat? Very possible says science researcher Gary Taubes, author of *Good Calories, Bad Calories*, who wrote:

> "The surge in obesity and diabetes occurred as the population was being bombarded with the message that dietary fat is dangerous and that carbohydrates are good for the heart and

weight control."[1]

Taubes, who is the only print journalist to have won three Science in Society awards given by the National Association of Science Writers, says;

> "This suggested the possibility, however heretical, that this official embrace of carbohydrates might have had unintended consequences…"[2]

Taubes is agreeing with Atkins that carbohydrates are the problem — "their effect on insulin secretion and thus the hormonal regulation of homeostasis."

> "It's quite possible that the low-fat, high carbohydrate diets we've been told to eat for the past thirty years are not only making us heavier but contributing to other chronic diseases as well."[3]

In his last book, *Age-Defying Diet Revolution*, Atkins takes final aim at "the Gospel according to the American Heart Association," which is, basically, avoid animal food, nothing else matters." Since 1961, the AHA has said:

🕊 Dietary fat — especially saturated fat — must be restricted.

🕊 Dietary cholesterol must be nearly eliminated.

🕊 Margarine and other polyunsaturated fats are heart-healthy.

🕊 Carbohydrates made with flour should be the basis of a healthy diet.

🕊 Eating 10 teaspoons of sugar a day is good for you.

In *Healthy Aging*, Andrew Weil, MD, says "For years, conventional doctors have focused obsessively on fat as the dietary culprit. They have told us to cut fat consumption drastically and have put countless people on low-fat diets without any regard for the amount and kinds of carbohydrate foods they were eating."[4]

Like Akins, Weil blames diabetes on carbohydrates — "the refined, quickly digested ones that place a high *glycemic* load on the system." Weil explains how "This pulverized starch is digested very rapidly, causing spikes in blood sugar and corresponding surges in insulin secretion…"[5]

In the chapter, "Why We Age," Weil writes, "Doctors have long observed accelerated development of a number of age-related diseases in people with diabetes, including cataracts and atherosclerosis. They also recognize that much of this pathology is the result of chemical reactions between glucose and proteins, a process called glycation…"[6]

As Atkins pointed out, "sugar is sticky." When you have elevated sugar or glucose in your bloodstream, those sticky glucose molecules can attach to protein. When glucose attaches to protein, it sets in motion a chain reaction of chemical reactions that ends with proteins slowly binding together, or cross-linking, and forming new chemical structures.

Glycation (or *glycosylation*) was discovered by biochemist, Anthony Cerami, Ph.D., National Academy of Sciences, as he observed patients with diabetes rapidly aging. He named these structures "advanced glycosylation end products," or AGEs. AGEs are dangerous because, in Atkins' words, "You're slowly cooking yourself from the inside."

Cross-linked proteins are less elastic, less flexible, and less able to perform their normal functions. Collagen, the primary building block of blood vessels, skin, lungs, and cartilage, is the first protein to be affected. After glycation, blood vessels stiffen, skin wrinkles, and joints can ache all over the body.

The link between accelerated aging and high blood sugar has been thoroughly documented. Clumps of cross-linked AGEs are found in the brains of people suffering with Alzheimer's, and, as doctors Atkins and Weil have both pointed out, cross-linked proteins cause cataracts in the eyes and promote "hardening" or calcification of the arteries.[7]

When AGEs latch on to low density lipoprotein (LDL), your body doesn't recognize the new substance as LDL and fails to clear it from the bloodstream. Diabetics — and those with pre-diabetes — have high levels of both oxidized LDL and glycated hemoglobin — damage to red blood cells from elevated blood sugar (A1c test)

Andrew Weil, MD, a vegetarian who eats fish and cheese, and the late Dr. Atkins, who considered animal foods healthy, have different philosophies about diet, but nonetheless agree that, as a society, we must reduce the percentage of carbohydrates and highly processed foods in our diets.

In *Healthy Aging*, Weil says:

> "That means less bread, white potatoes, crackers, chips and other snack foods, pastries and sweetened drinks… Less

refined and processed foods… Fewer products made with flour of any kind… no products listing partially hydrogenated oil… no vegetable shortening… do not eat margarine, regardless of what it is made from or what health benefits manufacturers claim for it…"[8]

These quickly digested carbohydrates and highly processed vegetable fats produce large numbers of free radicals — highly reactive out of balance molecules with one or more unpaired electrons. Excess free radicals promote advanced glycosylation end products, which, in turn, spike up free radical production.

Free radicals and AGEs deliver the one-two punches that cause us to age prematurely and die of heart disease, cancer and stroke, the leading causes of death. In Dr. Atkins' words:

"Avoiding, minimizing, and counteracting the damaging effects of free radicals must be the fundamental principle of any age-defying program."[9]

Published in the *Journal of the American Medical Association* (*JAMA*), February 25, 1998, the *Cardiovascular Health Study* followed 5,201 men and women age 65 or older for five years to answer the question, who lives longer and why:

"Elevated fasting blood sugar was one of the factors significantly and independently associated with mortality — blood cholesterol was not."

Study participants with higher LDL cholesterol — more than 153 mg/dl — had just two-thirds the mortality risk of participants with cholesterol less than 96 mg/dl, the supposedly desirable level. The Cardiovascular Health Study confirms what Atkins, Anthony Cerami, and Andrew Weil have been saying: Impaired blood sugar control damages blood vessels and accelerates aging.

According to Atkins, "Nearly half of all adults by the age of 50 will demonstrate at least some instability in their blood sugar and at least some insulin resistance."[10] In Andrew Weil's words, "High levels of sugar in the blood, even if transient, favor glycation and the production of compounds (AGEs) that damage body structures and distort its functions."[11]

According to Weil:

> "Even genetically sensitive people can minimize these problems by reducing the percentage of carbohydrates in their diet…"[12]

In 1973, Atkins was forced to defend himself before a congressional committee for promoting the same foods served to guests at George Washington's Mount Vernon. You don't get any more American than that! But this never stopped the American Heart Association from routinely attacking Atkins and labeling his diet a "dangerous fad."

Today, the American Heart Association's high carbohydrate diet is associated with record levels of obesity, diabetes, and heart failure. Though clearly wrong, the American Heart Association and the National Cholesterol Education Program continue to wage a decades-old Food War as tens of millions develop "diabesity" and die before their time.

Five Stages of Type 2 Diabetes

The first stage is *insulin* resistance, the common denominator of obesity, Type 2 diabetes, and heart disease. Insulin's job is to escort glucose into cells. In the carbohydrate-sensitive, in response to eating excess carbohydrates — especially boxed cereal and quickly digested carbohydrates — nutritionally deficit cells resist insulin.

When cells resist insulin, blood glucose levels rise. According to Dr. Atkins, insulin resistance is a consequence of intracellular mineral and vitamin deficiencies, especially magnesium, chromium, zinc, various trace minerals, and the B-complex vitamins.

Atkins refers to *Stage Two* as *hyperinsulinism*. Responding to high blood glucose, the pancreas floods the bloodstream with insulin. An overload of insulin forces some glucose into nutritionally deficient cells. According to Atkins, "The link between diabetes and heart disease begins at this stage."

Why? Because high blood insulin is *atherogenic* and can directly damage the *endothelial* cells lining artery walls, causing injury and inflammation that in time develops into plaque, blockage, and sticky, clot-prone blood.

In *Stage Three*, symptoms increase. Food cravings, brain fog, moodiness, fatigue, and irritability are brought on by hunger and relieved by eating — more carbohydrates. According to Atkins, the diagnosis of stage 3 requires a glucose tolerance test (GTT) which measures how the body uses blood sugar over a specific period of time. By the year 2000, Atkins had ordered this test for more than 40,000 of his patients.

Stage Four is Type 2 diabetes. Stages three and four are a continuum. Insulin resistance and hyperinsulinism rule but, in stage four, sugar remains elevated throughout the day. At this stage there are three must-have tests:

Test	Measures
Fasting glucose	Sugar in the blood after a 10 to 12 hour fast.
Postprandial test	How high your blood sugar and insulin go two hours after a high carb meal.
Hemoglobin A1c.	Average blood sugar over the past 2 or 3 months.

At *Stage Five*, the overworked pancreas finally crashes. At this final stage — full blown, insulin-dependent Type 2 diabetes, as in Type 1 diabetes, an external source of insulin is required.

In *Age-Defying Diet Revolution*, Atkins describes how blood vessel damage, sticky clot-prone blood, and the risk of heart attack increase throughout all five stages of Type 2 diabetes. Atkins wrote:

> "Excessive insulin, pre-diabetes, and refined carbohydrates have an awfully strong connection with shortening human life spans."[13]

> "Sugar is atherogenic — it causes heart disease. In addition to increasing levels of blood fats, such as blood triglycerides and the LDL to HDL ratio, sugar actually makes blood platelet cells…stickier and more likely to clump together."
> — *Burton Berkson, M.D.,* Syndrome X

More to Explore...

Well written detailed books about anti-aging

• *Dr. Atkins Age-Defying Diet Revolution* by Robert C. Atkins, MD. (New York: St Martin's Press, 2000). Dr. Atkins' final excellent book.

> "You'll learn the safest, surest ways to add many more years to your life, boost your immune defenses, enhance brain function, lose weight without restricting calories, combat Type 2 diabetes, and reduce the risk of cardiovascular disease."

• *The Modern Nutritional Diseases – and how to prevent them* by Alice and Fred Ottoboni, PhDs. (Sparks, NV: Vincente Books, 2002)

> "In this book, heart disease, stroke, type-2 diabetes and cancer are termed modern nutritional diseases because scientific studies and biochemical facts clearly point to the American Heart Association diet as a major underlying cause of these diseases. This so called heart-healthy diet outlined in the federal nutrition guidelines is based on faulty science. Sugar, starch and highly processed vegetable fat — not saturated fat and cholesterol — are responsible for high blood cholesterol, type-2 diabetes, and obesity."

• *Healthy Aging* by Andrew Weil, MD. (New York: Alfred A. Knopf, 2005)

> "Dr Weil's book about aging is unlike any other in the breadth and depth of its information and understanding — a lifelong guide to your physical and spiritual well-being."

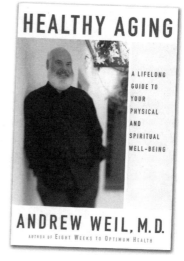

HEALTHY AGING

A LIFELONG GUIDE TO YOUR PHYSICAL AND SPIRITUAL WELL-BEING

ANDREW WEIL, M.D.

AUTHOR OF EIGHT WEEKS TO OPTIMUM HEALTH

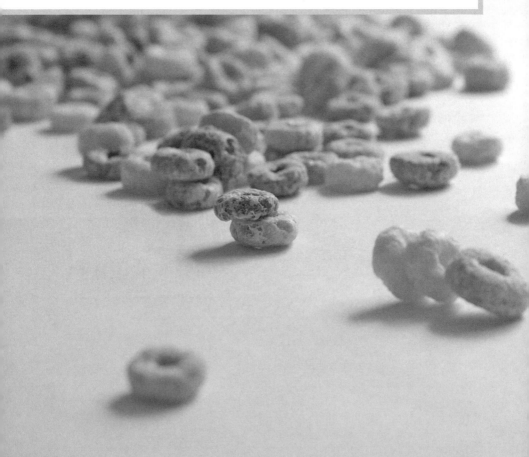

"High fructose corn syrup has no fiber or nutrients. While fructose doesn't raise blood sugar as fast as sugar, fructose raises triglycerides and actually increases insulin resistance, the root cause of Type II diabetes."

— *Journal of Nutrition, 1997, Vol. 127*

CHAPTER 4

Cereal Killer

"Members of the medical establishment
who continue to recommend sugar-laden
cereal as heart healthy should perhaps
be consulting with their attorneys."
— *Robert C. Atkins, M.D.*

Boxed cereals — refined or whole grain — tax our bodies with
what has been called "food chaos." According to Sally Fallon, author of
Nourishing Traditions cookbook, dry boxed cereals — those little flakes, o's,
puffs and animal shapes — are damaged by modern industrial extrusion.

As Fallon describes it: A wet slurry of grain — at very high
temperature — is forced out of little holes at very high pressure. After
extrusion, "A blade slices off each little puff or flake which is then carried
past a nozzle and sprayed with a coating of oil and sugar to make it go
crunch in milk."[1]

In *Fighting the Food Giants*, Paul Stitt says the extrusion process
destroys most of the nutrients in the grains.

> "It destroys the fatty acids; it even destroys the chemical
> vitamins that are added at the end. The amino acids are
> rendered very toxic by this process. The amino acid lysine,
> a crucial nutrient, is especially denatured by extrusion."[2]

All dry boxed cereals are made in this manner — even the dry boxed cereals sold in natural food groceries. Most Americans eat dry boxed cereal. In fact, the cereal companies gloat over the fact that most children today get their synthetic vitamins from dry boxed cereals. According to Kelloggs, "Pre-sweetened cereals, just like other cereals, provide many essential nutrients…"

But – don't forget the many grams of worthless sugar!

The highly touted whole grains are potentially more damaging than refined grains. Because whole grains contain more protein and protein is damaged the most by extrusion, dry boxed whole grains magnify "food chaos."

Paul Stitt describes an experiment carried out in the 1960s at the University of Michigan at Ann Arbor. Eighteen laboratory rats were divided into three groups:

🐭 One group received rat chow and water

🐭 A second group ate corn flakes and water

🐭 The third group ate the cardboard box and water

The rats eating rat chow and water remained in good health throughout the experiment. The rats eating the cardboard and water became lethargic and eventually died of malnutrition. The rats eating the corn flakes and water died first. Before death, the rats eating corn flakes developed schizophrenic behavior, threw fits and tantrums, bit at each other, and went into convulsions.[3]

Designed as a joke, this experiment may remind us of 4-year-old Bruce, biting other children until they bleed (see next chapter, "Class of 2018"). High sugar experiments are going on in millions of American households everyday. Popular children's cereals contain a lot of sugar and are usually doled out at twice the recommended serving. As one cereal manufacturer has advertised:

"It's not just for breakfast anymore!"

Another big problem with cereal is the milk. Indoor cows living on cement floors produce poor quality, watery milk — and live no more than a year! Cows are ruminants; good conscience and our mutual biology would have them back on pasture. (My grandfather's dairy cows lived up to 10 years and had names like "Betsy" over their stalls.)

Milk from these indoor "farms" is then shipped to large centralized factories where it is separated by centrifuge into fat, protein, and other solids and liquids. Oxidized dry milk powder is added back to the reduced fat milk to help restore flavor. This is the oxidized cholesterol we should be warned about — but are not!

Industrial "milk" is then pasteurized at 161 degrees — denaturing the proteins and destroying many nutrients, including vitamins C and B12. Like extruded cereals, pasteurized milk is heat-damaged and nutrient deficient. Homogenization is the final insult, destroying the fat by forcing it through tiny holes at high pressure and high temperature.

In *The Crazy Makers*, Carol Simontacchi describes how a sugary breakfast is harming children. Well meaning mothers set out breakfast cereal, skim milk, toast and orange juice for breakfast. Most children's cereals contain at least 15 grams (5 teaspoons) of sugar — in one serving. The cereal, milk sugar, toast, jam and orange juice rapidly digest down into simple sugar in the blood.

> "Such a load of blood sugar is dangerous for the brain. Although the brain is fueled by sugar, it can't handle excessive sugars so the pancreas leaps to the rescue, dumping insulin into the bloodstream to remove excess sugars before they can 'burn' the brain."[4]

In response to a sugary breakfast, large amounts of insulin are released. Just as rapidly, sugar is pulled from the blood into the liver. When the liver is full, the excess sugar is turned into fat, contributing to the rise in obesity.

As Simontacchi points out, "It might be better to give your kid a soft drink for breakfast than a bowl of breakfast cereal. Ounce per ounce, most breakfast cereals contain more sugar than soft drinks."[5]

Kids' Cereal	Serving/Size (grams)	Sugar (grams)	% Sugar	Protein (grams)	Fiber (grams)
Coco Roos	30	15	50	1	< 1
Cap'n Crunch	27	12	44	1	1
Cocoa Puffs	27	12	44	1	1
Froot Loops	30	13	43	1	1
Trix	32	13	40	1	1
Lucky Charms	27	11	40	2	1
Fruity Pebbles	30	11	36	1	3
Frosted Flakes	30	11	36	1	1

Dr. Robert Lustig, professor of pediatrics, University of California, says, "It's not one bowl of cereal. Most kids don't stop at one bowl." Lustig says high sugar at breakfast promotes hormonal imbalances that encourage kids to overeat. "More overweight children are developing diabetes, high cholesterol, and heart disease."[6]

Dr Lustig reminds us not to blame the victim, rejecting the common view that individual behavioral changes are all that is needed. "The reason [cereals] are so popular is that kids will pester their parents to buy them. You'll notice the sugared cereals are put down at eye level for children and there is a specific marketing strategy going on there."[7]

Lustig accuses the "big food companies" of aggressively marketing toxic food to children. Lustig emphasizes that human genetic make up hasn't changed over the last three decades, but the food processing industry has. Lustig links those changes to the rise in obesity and diabetes:

> "The high sugar content in foods and drinks and the decrease in fiber [and fat] create hormonal imbalances that actually cause people to eat more and exercise less."[8]

The most dramatic change in human diets in the past 10,000 years is the transition from a high fat hunter-gatherer diet to a high carbohydrate, grain-based diet that came with the invention of agriculture. During the last 100 years, we have witnessed the ever increasing refinement of those carbohydrates.

Per capita consumption of simple sugars increased from less than 10 or 20 pounds in the mid-eighteenth century to 150 to 160 pounds today. In the U.S. and throughout the world, we have seen a dramatic increase in grain, sugar and fructose consumption — all quickly digested carbohydrates

Relatively new to the human gut, grains can render many of us weak and bloated. Since grains can be difficult to digest, do not provide complete or optimum protein, and can raise blood sugar and insulin, many of us should avoid them altogether.

If you gain weight easily or if diabetes or heart disease "runs in your family," you must pay particular attention to your carbohydrate intake. People who consume more carbohydrate than their metabolism can handle are at risk of developing a cluster of risk factors called Metabolic Syndrome.

Coined "Syndrome X" by Dr. Gerald Reaven, Stanford University

Medical School, Metabolic Syndrome is pre-diabetes — chronic high blood sugar and high circulating insulin. Reaven estimates that at least 25 percent of us must restrict carbohydrates, even healthy-sounding whole grains. According to Reaven:

> "The Syndrome X culprit isn't red meat or butter, its carbohydrates."[7]

The anti-saturated fat dogma that grew out of the federal nutrition guidelines is coming back to haunt us. Grains have been emphasized — 6 to 11 servings per day — but grains provide incomplete protein and, when eaten in excess, put upward pressure on blood sugar, insulin and triglycerides in a deadly manner (see "Cholesterol is not a Medical Criminal," Chapter 8).

Although a high fat bacon and egg breakfast is the gold standard for complete protein, vegetarians and those who enjoy grains would benefit nutritionally by learning how to prepare the old fashioned whole grain porridges described in Sally Fallon's *Nourishing Traditions* cookbook.

While whole grains contain some highly touted *phytonutrients*, you must soak or sprout them in order to neutralize the *antinutrients*. Whole grains contain *phytate* in the outer layer or bran. Untreated, phytic acid can combine in the intestinal tract with calcium, magnesium, copper, iron, and especially zinc and block their absorption.[8]

According to Fallon, "These porridges should be soaked overnight in an acid medium to get rid of the anti-nutrients. Soaking will neutralize the tannins, complex proteins, enzyme inhibitors and phytic acid."[9]

> "You soak the grains in warm water with one tablespoon of something acidic like whey, yoghurt, lemon juice or vinegar. The next morning, the porridge cooks in about a minute. Of course, you eat your porridge with butter or cream like our grandparents did."[10]

The fat soluble vitamins A and D are needed to absorb the nutrients in the grains. That says Sally Fallon, was one of the great lessons of Weston A. Price, the Cleveland dentist who traveled around the world to study native people and learn about traditional foods. "Without the vitamins present in animal fats (vitamins A and D), you cannot assimilate minerals and other vitamins."

For optimum nutrition, its time to dust off our early 1900s cookbooks that provide recipes for a traditional high fat American diet emphasizing butter, cream, bacon, lard, raw milk, eggs, mutton, beef, pork, chicken, whole grain porridges, fruits in season, and great vegetable dishes lathered in luxuriant cream sauces.

American Hero: Weston A. Price (1870-1948)

In the early 1930s, Weston A. Price, a Cleveland dentist, began traveling to isolated parts of the world to study the health and diets of people eating traditional, non-Western diets. One stated purpose was to discover the factors responsible for good dental health. Already in the 1930s, in his Cleveland practice, Dr. Price noticed children with narrowed faces, crowded teeth, and excess dental carries.

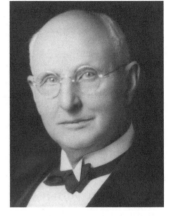

When Dr. Price analyzed the diets of native people eating traditional diets, he discovered that, in comparison to the American diet of his day, native diets provided at least four times the water-soluble vitamins (including calcium and other minerals), and at least ten times the fat-soluble vitamins (such as butter, fish eggs, organ meat, eggs and animal fats).

Dr. Price discovered that the abundant fat-soluble vitamins A and D were catalysts for mineral absorption and protein utilization. Without them, our bodies cannot absorb and utilize minerals. He also discovered a fat-soluble nutrient he called Activator X, now thought to be vitamin K2.

Best known as a nutrient for blood coagulation, new research indicates vitamin K is also required for healthy bones and blood vessels. Inadequate vitamin K may lead to calcification of the blood vessels and increased risk of heart disease. (Vitamin K in milk, what Price called Activator X — is destroyed by pasteurization.)

In a recent study in the Netherlands, researchers found, after correcting for age and other factors, that higher vitamin K2 reduced the risk of coronary heart disease mortality by 27 percent and severe aortic calcification by 29 percent. Vitamin K2 from meat, eggs, cheese and fermented foods was protective; vitamin K1 from dark-green leafy vegetables and vegetable oils was not.

The Price-Pottenger Nutrition Foundation was founded in 1952. The Foundation is independent of commercial interests and is dedicated to promoting and safeguarding the research and writings of Dr. Price.

They offer to the public and the healing professions vast historical and anthropological findings about traditional diets and up-to-date, accurate scientific information on nutrition and health. The Foundation is known for its integrity and accuracy in making this information available to the public.

More to Explore...

• *Nutrition and Physical Degeneration* by Weston A. Price. This is the classic study of Dr. Price's worldwide investigation of the deleterious effects of processed foods and synthetic farming methods on human health, First published in 1939, this book is as relevant today as it was 60 years ago.

This is the 2008 revised, expanded edition with a new cover and fifty-six new photographs never before seen in print. All of the photos have been restored and rescanned — the clearest photos ever published in this book. Also, new chapters with articles and correspondence to and from Dr. Price have been added.

The book includes Dr. Price's unforgettable photographs showing the superb dentition and facial development of people living on nutrient-dense foods. All who plan to bear children, everyone concerned about longevity, and those in the practice of medicine should read this book.

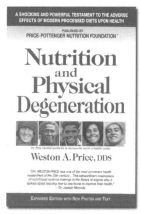

Available from the Price-Pottenger Nutrition Foundation by calling 800-366-3748 (in the US) or (619) 462-7600. Available online at www.ppnf.org.

527 pages, 196 photos, 6 maps,
softcover, $27.95

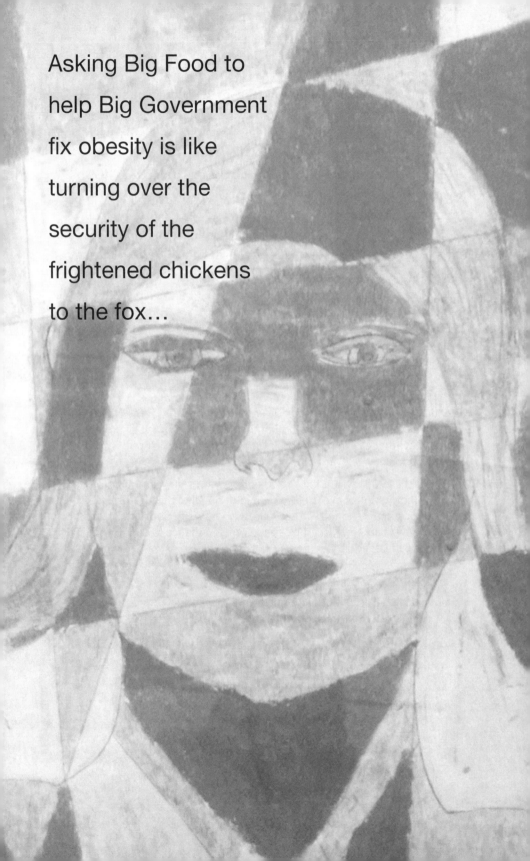

Asking Big Food to help Big Government fix obesity is like turning over the security of the frightened chickens to the fox...

CHAPTER 5

Class of 2018

"If the Center for Disease Control prediction is accurate, 45 to 50 million U.S. residents could have diabetes by 2050."
— *Dr. Kevin McKinney, University of Texas*

The headline reads: "Health Advisors To Battle Obesity in Children." "We call for action to be taken immediately, given the alarming rate at which the incidence of childhood obesity is growing in America," said Jeffrey Koplan, chairman of the committee.[1] Schools, parents, industry, and government must work together, he stressed.

While the increase in obesity can be seen across the country in all income and racial groups, the urban poor are affected the most. By the time they reach age 3, more than one-third of low-income children are overweight or obese, including 44 percent of low income Hispanic children.

Mark P. Becker, dean of the University of Minnesota School of Public Health, says obesity isn't a matter of individual choice or consequence. "There are significant societal costs — economic and otherwise — associated with the obesity epidemic."[2]

Becker, added:

> "A particularly alarming aspect of the obesity epidemic is that it is harming our children in significant numbers and in devastating ways. Type 2 diabetes, once considered an adult

disease, is now being diagnosed in children and teens as a direct result of the shocking increase in childhood obesity."[3]

The *Health Advisors'* recommendation to schools: "Make sure that all foods available are consistent with *federal nutrition guidelines...*" The *Health Advisors'* recommendation to the federal government: "Convene a task force to look at possible advertising restrictions. Include the food, beverage and entertainment industries."[4]

But, since 1980, schools have been required to meet federal nutrition guidelines. As for involving the food companies, they are already busy defending "their right" to advertise to children. According to the Minneapolis *Star Tribune*:

> "If Congress tries to restrict advertising, the industry will probably challenge it in court by arguing truthful speech is protected under the constitution."[5]

General Mills, Kelloggs and Kraft recently formed the "Alliance for American Advertising," a lobbying group to fight regulation of their ad practices. "Marketing to children is vital to these companies," says Dave Siegel, president of WonderGroup, a youth marketing agency that does business with General Mills, Kellogg's, and Kraft.[6]

According to the Institute of Medicine, food and beverage companies spend $10 to $12 billion a year advertising to children. Defending his company's advertising practices before the Institute's Committee on Food Marketing, Ken Powell, General Mills executive vice president, said:

> "Advertising is a crucial part of delivering innovation to our consumers."[7]

Or, is it delivering diabetes to children?

A record number of children in General Mills' target market already have Type 2 diabetes. According to the CDC, one in three American children born in the year 2000 will become diabetic. The odds are worse for black and Hispanic children, nearly half are at risk!

According to Gary Taubes, the incidence of diabetes began to increase dramatically in the 1980s as the number of overweight American children tripled during the first decade of "low fat." These young diabetics will die sooner and have a much higher lifetime risk of amputations, blindness, circulation problems, heart disease, and kidney failure.

Startled "health experts" are warning that obesity is driving up type 2 diabetes here and around the globe. The American Diabetes Association says there is no cure; only disease management with prescription drugs, insulin, and a "low fat" diet that emphasizes "carbohydrate choices" spread throughout the day.

Asthma is surging in children

Rita grew up in the 1960's knowing she was different. She ran out of breath often and struggled to breathe. Her parents and teachers said she was "high strung." It wasn't until she was in her late teens that Rita learned she had asthma. Now a mother of three, Rita has two sons with asthma.

Asthma is surging in children, especially black children. According to the CDC, blacks visit emergency rooms and are hospitalized and die of asthma three times the rate of whites.[8] The yearly cost of treating asthma has reached $11 billion with no end in sight.

A first diagnoses is often made during emergency room visits — 500,000 last year. In an attack, narrowed air passages are squeezed tighter. Common symptoms are wheezing, chest tightness, and shortness of breath. Attacks are triggered by allergies, dust mites, many common pollutants, and stress of all kinds.

According to a 2006 National Institutes of Health study, *steroidal inhalers* may have helped some high risk kids, but *"the study observed temporary slowing of growth in children using the steroids."*[9] There is now evidence, said Dr. Fernando Martiniz, University of Arizona, doctors were hasty in prescribing these inhalers to children under five.

Doctors may have to rethink their treatment options for children like Bruce. Born several weeks too soon, Bruce was a colicky baby who required a special formula until he was 10 months old. He experienced night terrors until age 3. By age 4, Bruce had hit another boy with a baseball bat and had bitten other children until they bled.

As he grew older, Bruce became more controlling. He was kicked out of several day care centers by age 6. His mom told case workers, "He has no sense of boundaries and rules." When angry, he smashes objects and flips over furniture in his path. He has defiantly smeared his feces on apartment walls and floors.

Recently, Bruce put a knife to his throat and threatened to kill himself. Deemed a threat to himself and his younger brother, Bruce was placed in foster care. His separated, unmarried parents have surrendered parental rights. Bruce's treatment: He is on *Ritalin*, *Effexor* and *Clonidine*.

But is anyone asking what Bruce had for breakfast?

What sugary cereal did he like best? Did Bruce's young mother consume enough saturated fat and cholesterol to make a healthy baby? How much corn syrup and hydrogenated fat had she been eating? Did she nurse Bruce or give him a soy formula loaded with high fructose corn syrup?

By feeding Bruce empty calorie, high sugar products like *Count Chocula* and *Froot Loops*, Bruce's mother was actually following federal nutrition guidelines, which, since 1980, have emphasized grain and grain products — like the sugary boxed cereals eaten daily in 93 percent of all American households.

Most American children are "growing up" on high fructose corn syrup, sugar, highly processed vegetable fats, a palette of food colors, and spray-on, synthetic vitamins. The "low fat" products that contain these cheap additives also contain double digit grams of refined flour and all too often the AHA "low fat" seal of approval.

"Low-fat diets are associated with greater feelings of anger, hostility, irritability, and depression. These mood changes appear to be biological consequences of inadequate dietary fat in the central nervous system."
—*British Journal of Nutrition*, 1998, Vol. 79

And, why are so many babies premature? Bruce was born at 26 weeks. (Most premature births are between 32 and 37 weeks.) Concerned health officials are reporting a 27 percent increase in premature births over the last 20 years — now 1 in 8. The rate for black mothers is almost 20 percent.[10]

Premature birth is the leading cause of developmental disability in children, including cerebral palsy and mental retardation. "None of the interventions used to try to reduce prematurity actually is effective," says Robert L. Goldenburg, professor in the department of obstetrics and gynecology at the University of Alabama.[11]

Asthma, obesity, diabetes, heart and reproductive failure are not contagious. The problem is what we are eating and what we are told to eat. In America, pet dogs and cats eat better than most children. The Class of 2018 is getting sicker, and the health and longevity of future generations depends, in part, on who grows our food and who revises the 2010 federal nutrition guidelines.

Isn't it finally time to ask, "Has *low fat* failed the test of time?" Could the millions of tons of hydrogenated vegetable fat and the billion boxes of sugary cereal served up during the last forty years be contributing to the big surge in asthma, obesity, Type 2 diabetes, and bipolar children like Bruce?

In Washington, DC, it's an uphill fight to protect children.

Iowa Democratic Senator Tom Harkin has accused General Mills and other cereal manufacturers of using cartoon characters like *Shrek* to encourage children to eat unhealthy products, but the big corporations and lobbying groups that oppose Harkin have a lot of clout in the Capital.

The American Heart Association has a lot of clout too. For decades, they've been collecting fees for awarding their "low fat" seal of approval to products like Yogurt Burst Cheerios, a dry boxed cereal that contain 9 grams of sugar in a 30 gram ¾ cup serving. Do the math. Yogurt Burst Cheerios are 30 percent sugar.

Now, why would a "heart association" recommend that we start our day with nine (9) grams of sugar — a metabolic toxin with no nutritional value — and then warn us away from eating an egg that contains less than ½ gram of cholesterol — a substance found in every cell in our bodies?

Yogurt Burst Cheerios	Eggs fried in butter
Two servings Yogurt Burst (no milk)	Two eggs (one tablespoon of butter)
4 grams of incomplete protein	14 grams of complete protein
18 grams of worthless sugar	No sugar
No valuable cholesterol	570 mg of cholesterol (¹/₂ is absorbed)
Raises blood sugar	Doesn't raise blood sugar
Calories: 240	Calories: 240

Please note: One milligram (mg) = 1/1000 of a gram

Aimed at children, Cookie Crisps contains 11 grams of sugar in a 26 gram ¾ cup serving. Yes — 40 percent sugar and one (1) gram of protein — the stuff young, growing bodies are supposed to be made of. But, that's okay, when the box is empty your child can make his or her own **Rocket Rider**! ("See side panel for assembly instructions.")

The first four ingredients in *Cookie Crisps* after whole grain corn:

Sugar

Brown Sugar

Corn meal

Chocolate flavored chips

According to science writer Gary Taubes:

> "Sugars — sucrose and high fructose corn syrup specifically — are particularly harmful… Through their direct effect on insulin and blood sugar, refined carbohydrates, starches, and sugars are the dietary cause of coronary heart disease and diabetes… By stimulating insulin secretion, carbohydrates make us fat and ultimately cause obesity."[12]

Don't look to Big Food for help! The food industry's fingerprints are all over the carbohydrate-based federal nutrition guidelines, and big companies like General Mills, Kellogg's, and Kraft are prepared to go to court to protect "market share" and their perceived "right" to advertise to children.

Dry Boxed Cereals = Blood-sugar raising "high glycemic" food products

Although excess refined carbohydrates deplete the body's mineral and nutrient reserves, all carbohydrates — including the more nutritious so called whole grains — raise blood sugar. The glycemic index (GI) ranks carbohydrates according to how fast they raise blood sugar. (Dietary fat and protein do not raise blood sugar or call for insulin.)

Foods that break down quickly during digestion score highest on the glycemic index and are referred to as "high glycemic." When you eat these foods, blood sugar increases rapidly. Even some healthy sounding carbohydrates have high glycemic values.

The glucose-based index rates baked potatoes at 98, parsnips at 97, and cooked carrots at 92. Although these numbers vary a little from index to index, starchy carbohydrates raise blood sugar much more quickly than low glycemic carbohydrates like broccoli and cauliflower (both rated under 40).

Rated at 51, a moderately glycemic sweet potato releases glucose more slowly than a baked potato (98). Rated at 49, old-fashioned Irish oatmeal is a better choice than Cream of Wheat, rated at 70. Both are better than highly processed boxed cereals that generally have high glycemic values.

Among fruits, dried dates (103) raise sugar faster than bananas (62), which raise sugar faster than apples (39), grapefruit (26), or cherries (23). While whole fruits vary in how fast they release sugar, they are always a healthier choice than concentrated fruit juices.

Food processing increases your body's glucose and insulin response. An apple is better than applesauce which is better than apple juice which is better than apple juice concentrate. Both fat and fiber slow glucose entry into the bloodstream.

The GI has complicating factors. Different types of potatoes and different processing or harvesting methods can influence glycemic values. As an example, cooked carrots raise blood sugar faster than raw carrots. The exact glycemic value of a banana can depend on how ripe it is. Canned beans release sugar faster than beans soaked and prepared at home.

In spite of the above, the GI is a useful guide that is especially helpful to people who are insulin resistant, diabetic or overweight. The GI would suggest to the carbohydrate sensitive that they avoid starchy vegetables and bread most of the time and eat their carrots raw.

Because the fiber in any flour is no longer intact, bread, bagels and muffins — whether made with whole wheat or white flour — are high glycemic. Whole wheat flour found in bread and cereals breaks down quickly and raises blood sugar just as fast as white flour products. Starchy foods have higher glycemic values than sugar, but foods that contain both sugar and starch are always high glycemic.

The glycemic index is just one way of assessing carbs. Carbohydrate density — the number of carbohydrate grams a food contains — must be considered. Beans may have moderate glycemic values, but they are carbohydrate dense and require a longer period of insulin release. Even with moderate

GI's, beans are too much carbohydrate for the carbohydrate-sensitive.

Nutritional value is important too. Refined white sugar may not raise blood sugar as fast as figs and dates, but sugar robs the body of vitamins and minerals while dates and figs have redeeming nutritional value. Don't let the lower glycemic rating of sugar overshadow the fact that sugar is worthless — no fiber or nutritional value.

The more whole grains, starchy vegetables and legumes you eat, the higher your overall insulin response. To spare insulin, carbohydrate sensitive individuals should emphasize low glycemic vegetables. They cause minimal rises in glucose, spare insulin, and have fewer digestible carbohydrates.

For most people most of the time, low glycemic carbohydrates have advantages over high glycemic foods. Rated below 40, broccoli, cauliflower, chick-peas, lentils, Lima beans, summer squash, and zucchini are slow releasers.

Dietary fats brake rising blood sugar in two ways. Fat is digested more slowly than carbohydrates, and eating fat and protein at each meal reduces the amount of carbohydrate eaten — lowering the meal's glycemic load.

Butter on bread, butter and sour cream on baked potato, or butter, cream, and milled flaxseed in oatmeal will slow the sugar release of the meal. Most dry boxed cereals raise insulin; lamb chops, herring, and eggs won't.

To curb weight gain and reverse obesity, emphasize protein, fat, and a variety of low glycemic vegetables, smothered in rich cream sauces! It's that simple! High glycemic carbohydrates and excess carbohydrates — especially sugars and starches — raise blood sugar and insulin levels and promote elevated triglycerides (Tg), a major risk factor for heart disease (see Chapter 8).

The glycemic index shown below uses glucose as the reference index and are compiled from various sources, including *Syndrome X* (by Jack Challem, Burton Berkson, MD, and Melissa Diane Smith); *Dr. Atkins Age-Defying Diet Revolution*; *Genetic Nutritioneering* by Jeffrey S. Bland, Ph.D.; and Glycemic Index Lists at www.mendosa.com. For a complete online listing, go to www.glycemicindex.com.

High-Glycemic Foods

- Whole wheat and white bread
- Boxed breakfast cereals (most)
- Instant/quick cooking cereals and grains
- Grain-based snack foods/chips
- Honey and table sugar
- Cookies, cakes, and candy bars
- Potatoes, especially baked
- Dates/other dried fruits
- Brown and white rice
- Cooked carrots
- Pizza
- Waffles and donuts
- Crackers

Moderate-Glycemic Foods

- Yams and sweet potatoes
- Kidney beans (canned)
- Slow cooking oatmeal
- Pinto and navy beans
- Green peas
- Bananas
- Beets
- Sweet corn

Low-Glycemic Foods

- Asparagus, broccoli and cauliflower
- Chinese cabbage (bok choy)
- Celery, cucumber
- Green and red cabbage
- Chickpeas
- Lentils, black-eyed peas
- Fresh-cooked kidney beans

Low-Glycemic Foods *(continued)*

ꙮ Yellow and green beans

ꙮ Peppers

ꙮ Milk/yogurt

ꙮ Salad greens of all types

ꙮ Peanuts

ꙮ Spinach

ꙮ Zucchini and summer squash

More to Explore...

Recommended books about the food industry.

• Carol Simontacchi, *The Crazy Makers* (New York: Penguin Putnam, 2000)

"An unprecedented and impeccably reported look at how American food manufacturers and their products may be driving us crazy."

• Kaayla T. Daniel, PhD, *The Whole Soy Story* (Washington, DC: New Trends Publishing, 2005)

In this detailed, heavily referenced expose, Dr. Kaayla Daniel exposes "the dark side of America's so-called favorite health food. Hundreds of epidemiological, clinical and laboratory studies link eating highly processed soy to malnutrition, digestive problems, thyroid dysfunction, cognitive decline, reproductive disorders, immune system breakdown — and even heart disease and cancer."

• Ron Schmid, ND, *The Untold Story of Milk* (Washington, DC: New Trends Publishing, 2003)

"Ron Schmid details the betrayal of public trust by government health officials and dissects the modern myths concerning cholesterol, animal fats, and heart disease."

Andrew Weil, MD,
commenting on Gary Taubes' book, *Good Calories, Bad Calories* on *Larry King Live*, "Are Fatty Foods Good For You?" aired October 19, 2007

Dr. Weil: I think this is a very important book. I have been recommending it to my medical colleagues and students. He [Taubes] raises big questions and I think there are some very big ideas in this book:

"One of them is that there is absolutely no scientific evidence for the belief that fat is the driver of obesity."

"Secondly, the idea that it is carbohydrate which is central to this process and that obesity is mostly a hormonal disorder, genetically influenced, in which insulin is a central player."

"That overeating and under activity are not causes of obesity, but symptoms of that underlying disorder."

"It's not that people eat too much and don't exercise because of some defect of will or some behavioral problem; it's that this is behavior that is controlled by a hormonal disturbance."

"And I think he's done a meticulous job of showing that many of the assumptions that are held by the conventional medical community simply rest on nothing — that there's no scientific evidence for...."

http://transcripts.cnn.com/TRANSCRIPTS/0710/19/lkl.01.html

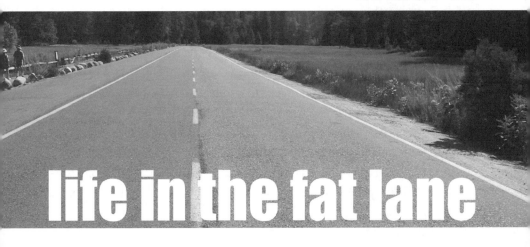

PART II

life in the fat lane

"Eating protein increases energy and keeps energy balanced throughout the day. One of the main causes of fatigue in many people, particularly women, is that they are not eating enough protein in the morning and at lunch."

— *Robert Crayhon, M.S.,* The Carnitine Miracle

"Earth Be Glad Farm"

A growing number of Minnesotans have become acquainted with Earth-Be-Glad Farm, nestled along the bluffs in southeastern Minnesota near Winona. The farm is located at the head of "Rupprecht's Valley," settled by Mike Rupprecht's great-great grandfather in 1860.

Mike, his wife Jennifer, and daughter Johanna operate a traditional family farm dedicated to healthy soil and healthy animals. They are busy maintaining pastures and raising grass-fed beef, chickens, and eggs without resorting to pesticides, antibiotics, growth hormones or genetic engineering.

If you drive by the farm when there's no snow on the ground, you will see pastures divided into paddocks so that the cattle can move daily to a lush "salad bar." This carefully managed grazing system provides the least possible negative impact on the environment.

Planned grazing builds up the soil as grass and roots grow and decay, while animal manure fertilizes pastures. This imitates the prairie ecosystem in which the great herds of buffalo existed. Earth-Be-Glad Farm has virtually no soil erosion and uses very little fossil fuel.

The Rupprecht's have experimented with native prairie species in some paddocks, and they always leave a paddock or two un-grazed for ground-nesting birds such as bobolinks. They increase biodiversity by seeding as many as 15 plant species in the pasture. The farm has tree lines and "edges" for nesting habitat for grassland birds and wildlife.

A walk through the pasture in May will reveal as many as 25 species of birds. The Rupprechts have noted the return of the eastern kingbird, Baltimore oriole, and several pair of bluebirds. A favorite, the brown thrasher, is the singing clown in the treetops.

The Rupprechts do not want to compromise the health of the soil and ecosystem by tilling the pasture for any other purpose — whether rows of crops or organic vegetables. They feel that permanent well-managed pasture is the best use of this highly erodible land and livestock are essential in improving soil fertility and stability.

Their cattle provide the rich manure and nitrogen-bearing urine for the replenishment of the soil. Mike checks on the pastured cattle twice each day, making sure that the water lines and fences are working properly. Mike, Jennifer and Johanna enjoy watching the young calves playing tag.

In the winter, the cattle are out on pasture when weather permits. Cattle are very adaptable to cold weather, but Mike takes extra care to provide wind protection. No artificial growth-promoting hormones, routine antibiotics or animal by-products are used. "Unknowns" are avoided to help assure that healthy meat can be part of your healthy diet.

The beef are finished on pasture and hay — no grains! — nature's design for ruminant animals. Research has shown that beef finished exclusively on forages has increased levels of omega 3 fatty acids, vitamin E, and CLA (conjugated linoleic acid).

The dreaded E.coli bacteria are lower in grass-fed beef because the ruminants are eating the forages their bodies were designed to eat. Commercial animals are force-fed a high grain diet that causes their systems to produce higher E. coli — which is then increasingly present in the meat.

Bypassing much of the conventional food system which is increasingly controlled by corporate giants, the Rupprecht's are working toward a new consumer paradigm in which the buyer of food knows the producer of food. Dealing face to face, the buyer provides a living for the producer and the producer provides nutritious food for the buyer.

Buy direct from farmers like the Rupprechts and you're getting their dedication to environmentally responsible farming, the humane treatment of animals, and an old fashioned respect for the future of the land. Your beef will be processed at a local plant, properly aged, and then packaged and frozen according to your specifications.

You can find Earth-Be-Glad Farm and other pastured products in your area online at www.eatwild.com and www.minnesotagrown.com.

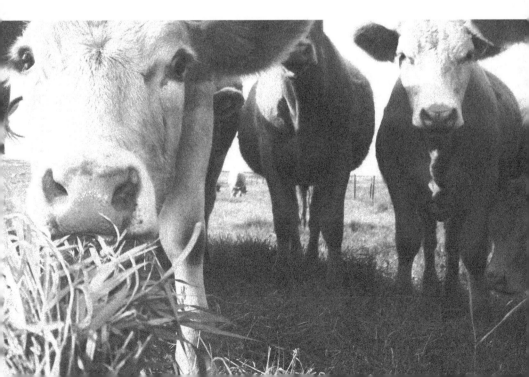

"In one study, researchers found that, way above whether patients had high cholesterol, the progression of plaque accumulation in the arteries was really due to elevated homocysteine. But even though high homocysteine has been known for decades to accelerate the risk of heart attack, stroke, macular degeneration, and Alzheimer's, many cardiologists don't check it. Since there is no drug treatment for homocysteine (the treatment is vitamins), the test is not very popular."

— *Sherry A. Rogers, M.D.*

CHAPTER 6

'Loose Lips Sink Ships'

"In the world of cardiovascular research, you cannot have a reputation if you dare to question the cholesterol hypothesis. You would be almost certainly cast instantly into the outer darkness."
— *Malcolm Kendrick, M.D.*

For decades in the U.S., the cholesterol theory, the idea that saturated fat and cholesterol clog arteries and cause heart attacks, has reigned supreme. Any doctor who challenged the fat and cholesterol hypothesis — as Atkins did — was ignored, ridiculed, persecuted, and "cast instantly into the outer darkness."

Since the inception of "cholesterol-is-to-blame," many researchers took issue with Ancel Keys' slippery science and continued to search for a better explanation. After all, many studies — especially Framingham — had not produced any convincing evidence that saturated fat and cholesterol were the cause of any disease.

In 1969, Dr. Kilmer McCully, a highly regarded physician at Harvard University and Massachusetts General Hospital, announced a significant medical breakthrough: The risk of heart attack and stroke were strongly associated with elevated levels of homocysteine, an amino acid metabolite produced in the body.

McCully published his findings in the *American Journal of Pathology*. According to McCully, elevated homocysteine was the underlying cause of heart disease — not cholesterol. B-vitamin deficiencies were to blame — not red meat. McCully concluded that elevated cholesterol and clogged arteries were secondary symptoms of heart disease — not causes.[1]

McCully's paper included a simple solution: Excess homocysteine is quickly removed from the bloodstream by restoring optimum levels of vitamins B6, B12 and folic acid. Plant and animal whole foods rich in B-vitamins are the cure, but nutritional supplements also reduce elevated homocysteine to lower levels.[2]

Already partners with the AHA on the cholesterol bandwagon, the National Institutes of Health (NIH) responded to McCully's paper by cutting off his funding. Harvard wasn't ready to challenge the cholesterol hypothesis either. McCully's research assistants were reassigned and he was asked to relocate to a basement office.

McCully was a graduate of Harvard College and Harvard Medical School. He had worked at Harvard for 16 years. He was in mid-career, had two children in college, and was now being forced to accept a drastically reduced income.

"To say that McCully's ideas were unwelcome at the cholesterol feast in the late 1970s would be a mammoth understatement," wrote *New York Times* reporter Michelle Stacey. "Many people had invested heavily in the cholesterol theory and few wanted to hear it challenged."[3]

Stacey asked, "Who exactly was it who had so much to lose if cholesterol took a back seat?" The answer came from Thomas N. James, cardiologist and president of the University of Texas Medical School. "It's the money that's a problem," he said. "Look at the colorful advertisements in general interest publications explaining to grandfather that his grandchildren want him to stay alive using these drugs…."[4]

> "The anti-cholesterol medications are multibillion dollar industries and they have a huge stake in fanning the flames of the cholesterol mission."[5]

After initially fighting for his job, McCully left Harvard to look for work, but "poison phone calls" made if difficult for him to get a second job interview anywhere in the country. After a corner-office Boston attorney put a stop to the calls, McCully was offered a position at the Veterans Hospital in Providence, Rhode Island.[6] It wasn't Harvard, but McCully could continue his research.

Meanwhile, throughout the 1980s, researchers around the world were busy validating McCully's findings. At Harvard's School of Public Health, Meir Stampfer, M.D., professor of epidemiology and nutrition, evaluated homocysteine levels in the Physicians' Health Study, a 10-year survey of 15,000 doctors between the ages of 40 and 84.

In 1992, Stampfer and his researchers reported:

> The physicians with the highest blood homocysteine levels were three times more likely to have a heart attack than those with the lowest levels — but even mild elevations were associated with increased risk of heart disease.[7]

The Harvard study demonstrated that elevated homocysteine was not only an independent risk factor for heart disease, but also a much more predictive risk factor than cholesterol. According to Dr. Stampfer:

> "The majority of heart attacks occurred in individuals with 'normal' cholesterol."[8]

Looking at Framingham data, Dr. Jacob Selhub, Tufts University, found a strong association between elevated homocysteine and low levels of vitamins B6, B12, and folic acid. According to Selhub, "The higher the homocysteine in the blood, the higher the prevalence of stenosis," the narrowing of the carotid artery leading to the brain.[9]

In a long-term study of 2,000 residents in western Jerusalem, elevated homocysteine was linked to heart disease and all causes of death. Trial participants with mild to moderately elevated homocysteine had a 30 to 50 percent greater risk of death compared to those with the lowest levels.[10]

"Elevated homocysteine aggravates all other mechanisms involved in atherosclerosis," wrote the late Dr. Atkins. "High homocysteine is an almost uncanny alarm bell that signals an increased danger of vascular disease, whether coronary, peripheral, or cerebral."[11]

Shunned for two decades, McCully was back in the limelight in Ireland at the first International Conference on Homocysteine in 1995. Introduced as the "father of homocysteine," McCully was acknowledged as the first researcher in the world to make the homocysteine-heart disease connection.

Even his former detractors in the American Heart Association were forced to agree that homocysteine warranted further study. Showing no bitterness, McCully added, "I thought it was great that these big shots were finally paying attention to it." McCully quietly supports the "follow-the-money" explanation for what happened to him at Harvard:

> "People don't make a profit preventing disease," he says. "They make a profit through medicine—treating critically advanced stages of disease."[12]

In 1997, McCully published *The Heart Revolution* (published in 1999 as *The Homocysteine Revolution*). McCully wrote, "Deficiencies of B vitamins in the diet — folic acid, vitamin B6 and vitamin B12 — trigger heart disease by raising the level of homocysteine in the blood."[13]

And McCully added:

> "The previously touted dangers of dietary fats and cholesterol need to be reconsidered… the millions of research dollars spent trying to prove the cholesterol theory have all come up empty-handed."[14]

Homocysteine is a normal byproduct of metabolizing methionine, an essential amino acid the body uses to build muscle. Homocysteine is usually rapidly cleared from the bloodstream, but when there are B-vitamin deficiencies, homocysteine will build up in the blood and cause damage to tissues.

(Biochemical processes usually require enzymes or cofactors. The cofactors required to convert homocysteine to one of its nontoxic cousins — methionine or cysteine — are the three B-complex vitamins, B6, B12 and folic acid.)

According to McCully, high homocysteine is also a consequence of advancing age, high blood sugar, diabetes, smoking, certain prescription drugs, hypertension, and hormonal changes such as menopause.[15]

A homocysteine reading of more than 8 micromoles per liter means increased risk of heart disease. Risk is linear; the higher your homocysteine, the greater the risk. Homocysteine levels above 14 increase your risk of heart attack and stroke two to four times.

When elevated, homocysteine promotes clotting and is a serious risk factor for clotting not just in the coronary arteries but also in the veins and arteries in the legs and in the carotid artery leading to the brain.[16]

Elevated homocysteine is even more dangerous when it's associated with other clotting risk factors, and multiple risk factors may be especially dangerous for people who have recently undergone invasive vascular treatments like heart bypass operations, stents or balloon angioplasty.[17]

In the long run — in terms of your overall health — your best option is to replace refined, enriched foods with whole foods, plant and animal.

- ✞ Liver and other organ meats are the best sources of vitamins B6, B12, and folic acid. Liver and organ meats from pasture raised animals are safe and excellent to eat on a regular basis.

- ✞ Food sources of vitamin B6 include liver, fish, red meat, poultry, peas, nuts, broccoli, Brussels sprouts, lentils, kale and properly prepared whole grains and beans.

- ✞ Food sources of vitamin B12 include liver, fish, red meat, cheese, raw milk, clams, oysters and eggs. (There are no reliable plant sources of B12. Soy foods increase the body's B12 requirement.)

- ✞ Excellent food sources of folic acid include liver and other organ meats, green leafy vegetables, grapefruit, nuts, peas and properly prepared whole grains and beans.

- ✞ Excess coffee per day (more than 2 cups) may increase homocysteine. Tea, which contains less caffeine, has little or no affect on homocysteine levels.

- ✞ Supplemental vitamin B6 (50-100 mg), folic acid (800-1,600 mcg), and vitamin B12 (1,000-2,000 mcg) quickly reduce elevated homocysteine. In the liver, by a separate enzymatic pathway, choline and betaine convert homocysteine to methionine. Derived from lecithin, choline is abundant in eggs and betaine is abundant in beets.

Eat eggs — not boxed cereal — for breakfast

Eating eggs — the gold standard for high quality protein — is a better way to start your day than loading up on sugary, heat-damaged, dry boxed cereal. If there is a perfect food, eggs would top the list.

Eggs contain all 8 essential amino acids, which are the building blocks of protein. Eggs are also a good source of the sulfur-containing amino acids (methionine, cysteine, and cystine) important for antioxidant protection and detoxification.

Eggs are the best dietary sources of phosphatidylcholine, also known as lecithin. Lecithin is a protector of every cell in the body and is the source for choline. Choline is a B-vitamin-like nutrient that also helps lower elevated homocysteine.

Eggs are the most concentrated source of the antioxidants lutein and zeaxanthin. Lutein and zeaxanthin form a yellowish deposit in the macula, the sensitive light-gathering area at the back of the eye. Without these antioxidants, blue and ultraviolet light can cause macular degeneration, the leading cause of blindness among people over 50.

Over 15 million Americans already have macular degeneration. In his newsletter, the late Dr. Robert C. Atkins, asked:

> "Can you just imagine how much macular degeneration could have been prevented if eggs yolks hadn't been seen as the dietary enemy for so long?"

Eggs also provide folic acid, vitamin B6, and vitamin B12—nutrients that prevent homocysteine buildup in the blood. Other nutrients in eggs include "heme" iron, magnesium, calcium, potassium, zinc, trace minerals, and vitamins A, D, E, and K.[19]

Decades ago, the Cereal Institute, a member of the National Cholesterol Education Program, sponsored a trial in which they gave volunteers "dry egg powder." Dry egg powder contains oxidized cholesterol and is harmful to your health. No one should eat dry egg powder. Can you believe this is the only study that condemned eggs decades ago?

What do highly processed boxed cereals have to offer? Do they contain any naturally occurring lutein, zeaxanthin, choline, methionine, cysteine, cystine, vitamin B6, or vitamin B12? Hardly — but most contain a lot of sugar. When you pour skim milk on boxed cereals, you are adding milk sugar to refined sugar to grain sugar. You'll get your sugar all right — high fasting glucose, insulin resistance, and diabetes.

Boycott those highly processed, heat damaged Puffs, Charms, Circles, Flakes, and Pops. Instead, eat fresh brown eggs for breakfast—as many as you like—poached, scrambled, or fried slowly in butter or lard.

Cage-free, small producer eggs are best — richer in fat-soluble vitamins A, D, E and K and the unsaturated long-chain omega 6 and omega 3 essential fatty acids. Most important, small producer eggs from pasture-fed chickens contain a 1:1 ratio of omega 6 to omega 3 – in contrast to the adverse 20:1 ratio found in the eggs from grain-fed commercial caged-up chickens.

High quality eggs are health promoting. You can eat them everyday in a variety of ways. They're especially important for growing children. If you've been stuck in the oatmeal or Cheerios rut, get crackin'!

Author's Note:

Throughout *Cereal Killer*, when I am recommending beef, chicken, eggs, bacon, lard, and dairy products, I am referring to animals raised humanely — the old fashioned way. To the extent possible, it's also a good idea to make sure that your fruits, vegetables, and grains are free of antibiotics, pesticides, and other harmful chemicals.

More to Explore...

• Kilmer McCully, MD, *The Heart Revolution* (New York: HarperCollins Publishers, 1999). Published more recently as *The Homocysteine Revolution*.

Weight-loss doctor dies at 72 from head injuries

By Robert Davis, *USA TODAY*

"Cardiologist Robert Atkins, the weight-loss guru who put steak back on the nation's menu, died Thursday in New York from head injuries he suffered last week in a fall. He was 72.

Atkins fell and hit his head while walking to his office April 8, a day after a spring storm iced sidewalks. Surgeons removed a blood clot, but he lapsed into a coma.

A brash and controversial figure, Atkins was famous for his best-selling books touting a diet that included eggs, cheese, and meat. He was criticized for decades by doctors who favor a low-fat approach.

Atkins death comes as the medical establishment appears to be seeing him in a new light. Recent studies have found that people on the Atkins diet lost weight without compromising their health...."

CHAPTER 7

Atkins...without Atkins

"I am not a proponent of the Atkins diet, but I think we have to thank Dr. Atkins for drawing our attention to the role of carbohydrates in obesity."
— *Andrew Weil, M.D.*

Dr. Robert C. Atkins

Since 1961, we have been told in a million messages that dietary fat is the big issue in weight control. Food advertising, nutrition education, medical advice, food labels, textbooks, and weight loss programs all say: "Fear fat." With obesity surging, what do our experts recommend?

Quit eating while you're still hungry! Order an appetizer and share it with another dieter. Your protein serving should resemble a little deck of cards. Drink fat free milk. Use fat free salad dressings. Eat four pieces of fruit everyday (how bears fatten up for winter).

Don't expect any help from the 2005 federal nutrition guidelines. Nothing is more confusing and counter-productive than the calorie-counting weight loss recommendations. The government guidelines are based on, "A calorie is a calorie is a calorie." Fat people are fat because they eat too many calories and don't exercise enough:

> "An *energy imbalance* (more calories consumed than expended) is the most important factor contributing to the increase in overweight and obesity in this country."[1]

This is repeated so often it sounds true. It's on cereal boxes and in college textbooks. Dietitians say restrict fat (it's highest in calories), count your calories, and choose up to 65 percent of them as fruits, vegetables and grains. To help make this work, exercise your butt off 60 to 90 minutes a day.

If you have semi-starved yourself on one of these "eat less" calorie-counting programs, this chapter is for you. The fact that a high fat Atkins style diet could be more effective for fat loss may seem puzzling because fat gives off more calories when burned in a simple furnace-like device called a *bomb calorimeter*:

🌶 A gram of carbohydrate yields 4.2 calories (actually kilocalories or kcals).

🌶 A gram of protein produces 5.25 kcals — reduced to 4.25 kcals. (one calorie is deducted for urea and other protein byproducts)

🌶 A gram of fat yields 9.2 kcals.

Fat must be fattening, right? The answer is "no" when you look into this further. "To assume the human body, an almost infinitely complex dynamic system, works like an ordinary furnace or bomb calorimeter is to greatly oversimplify," says Fred and Alice Ottoboni, PhD's, authors of *The Modern Nutritional Diseases*.[2]

First, the primary function of dietary protein is making cells, tissues, organs, skin, blood, muscle, and hair. In well fed people on a high natural fat diet, protein calories are a secondary fuel and do not contribute much to the body's immediate caloric or energy needs.

Fat is a premium animal (and human) fuel — and is also used to replenish cell membranes and to provide building blocks for a wide range of biochemicals, including hormones and sheathing for the brain and nervous system. Much of our fat calories are used for "homeland security" — policing what goes in and out of cells.

🌶 Carbohydrates = mostly fuel/energy

🌶 Protein = construction and repair; secondary fuel

🌶 Fat = homeland security; premium fuel

Also (and briefly), if you emphasize fat and restrict carbohydrates, your body goes into mild *ketosis*, a normal, important energy pathway in animal biochemistry. Once in ketosis, much more energy (calories) is excreted — lost in urine and feces — than on high carbohydrate diets. The difference is nearly 3-fold according to studies by Alan Kekwick and Gaston Pawan cited by Taubes in *Good Calories, Bad Calories*.[3]

> "For healthy people on low carbohydrate diets, the only result of ketone body production is loss of body fat."[4]

Common sense should tell us that calories from carbohydrate add up differently than calories from protein and fat. But in government and medicine, "a calorie is a calorie is a calorie" and no one can prove otherwise! As Taubes put it:

"Low fat guidelines have become gospel."

In 1972, Dr. Robert C. Atkins, cardiologist and general practitioner, wrote:

> "The calorie counting approach has failed. Orthodox medicine's conspicuous lack of success in treating overweight hasn't caused the profession to search widely for alternatives…."[5]

In 2001, Walter Willett, M.D., professor, Harvard University, wrote:

> "In the United States, the gradual reduction in the fat content of the average diet from 40 percent of calories to about 30 percent has been accompanied by a gradual increase in the average weight and a dramatic increase in obesity."[6]

As Willett points out in the chapter, "Surprising News About Fat, "the average American has substantially reduced the percentage of calories that she or he gets from fat over the past three decades." Willett adds, "But we aren't any healthier for all of this effort. In fact, we're worse off for it."[7]

Dr. Atkins' clinical success treating obesity and Harvard's long-term population studies all suggest that carbohydrates are the problem and restricting them is the solution. There's plenty of evidence going back more than a century to show that sugars, grains, fruit and fruit juices raise blood sugar and promote fat storage in adipose tissue.

As a director of fat storage, insulin converts excess glucose into body-made-fat. When insulin levels are elevated — chronically or after a high carb meal — we accumulate fat in our tissues. By stimulating insulin and driving fat accumulation, carbohydrates increase hunger. (Trapped in storage, fat is not an available fuel to the rest of the body.)

In particular, it's the poor quality carbohydrates — especially white sugar and high fructose corn syrup — that overload the liver and cause excess fat accumulation in our tissues — not the total number of calories we consume. But all carbohydrates — including beans and whole grains — raise blood sugar and elevate insulin.

To burn fat, try restricting sugar, fructose, corn sweeteners, soft drinks, pastries, donuts, pies, most bread, bagels, boxed cereals, breakfast bars, soy milk, French fries (unless fried in animal tallow), white rice, rice cakes, jams, jellies, pancakes, puddings, sweet deserts, and most fruits, juices and so called smoothies.

The reason for restricting sugars and grains is to keep blood sugar and insulin in an optimum range. (Not a bad idea, huh?) Your main source of energy must come from fat. This fat-loss way of eating means you are replacing carbohydrates with fat. The Atkins' diet resembles George and Martha Washington's high fat diet.

In his best selling *Diet Revolution*, Atkins wrote, "I suddenly realized, seeing myself in a photograph, that I had three chins." Atkins began researching the medical literature to learn what he could do to lose weight and regain his vital energy:

> "I came upon some important information from the late
> Dr. Alfred W. Pennington, of the DuPont Company, who
> postulated that overweight is frequently explained by an
> intrinsic metabolic defect. He suggested a treatment for it that
> does not restrict calories."[8]

Dr. Pennington was hired by the DuPont Company after WW II to find out why low-calorie diets had failed with so many of their staff members. Pennington discovered that overweight could be caused not by overeating but by an inability of the body to utilize carbohydrates for anything except:

Making fat!

Twenty DuPont staff members volunteered to try Pennington's high fat carbohydrate restricted diet — eliminating sugar, cereal, and starch. No calorie counting. On the contrary, the diet allowed 3,000 calories a day, but anyone who was hungry was free to eat protein and fat without limit.

Throughout the test period, all twenty of Pennington's dieters reported they felt well and were never hungry. After three and one-half months, the participants had lost an average of 22 pounds. Those who had high blood pressure "discovered happily that it had dropped, parallel to their drop in weight."

In 1963, having thoroughly researched Pennington's results, Atkins decided to try what he called a "hungry man's diet."

> "When I started being my own guinea pig, I knew I was going to eat a lot of food and felt that I would be lucky to lose three or four pounds in a month. I was truly surprised — in fact it was probably the greatest surprise of my life — when at the end of six weeks on this diet I had lost twenty-eight pounds!"[9]

Atkins would say: Don't go hungry. Eat as much high quality protein and natural fat as your body tells you it needs. Just restrict your carbohydrates to no more than 50 to 72 grams per day. (The range, of course, accounts for individual differences.) By restricting excess carbohydrates, your body will burn fat — including the stored fat you want to lose.

Instead of starving fat off, burn it off!

Eat as much as you want of any quality meat, fish (without mercury), poultry, raw milk cheese, cream, butter and eggs. Emphasize naturally raised animal protein. Also, as Atkins did, eat avocados, berries, Brussels sprouts, broccoli, cabbage, cauliflower, celery, green leafy vegetables, kale, mushrooms, nuts, onions, spinach, tomatoes, etc. (up to 72 grams).

Atkins' clinical success was recognizing that high blood sugar and high insulin are associated with accelerated aging, cancer, high blood pressure, obesity, type 2 diabetes, and polycystic ovary syndrome. As Atkins was at pains to point out, when insulin levels are stabilized, you're protecting yourself from all of these conditions.

Why, then, would anyone in the medical and health professions encourage diabetics — or anyone for that matter — to emphasize carbohydrates, even if, as instructed by registered dietitians and nurse educators, they *"spread out their carbohydrate choices throughout the day?"*

In one of his last newsletters, Atkins wrote:

> "I don't think it requires a medical degree to know that diabetics have a problem with glucose and that high blood glucose levels make it worse. From the time blood-sugar levels could be tested, doctors knew that carbohydrate foods raised blood-glucose levels and non-carbohydrate foods would not."

In *Dr Atkins' Diet Revolution* (1972), Atkins expressed his outrage that the medical profession and health authorities were choosing to ignore the uniquely fattening role of carbohydrates. A high fat diet remained an important component of his distinguished 40 year career as a family doctor and cardiologist.

In April 2003, at age 72, while walking to his NY City office during a late winter storm, Atkins slipped on ice and hit the back of his head. Surgeons removed a blood clot, but he died in a coma one week later. According to *USA Today:*

> "Atkins' death came as the medical establishment appears to be seeing him in a new light. Recent studies have found that people on the Atkins diet lost weight without compromising their health."[10]

If you have fat to burn, do Atkins… without Atkins!

Recent Harvard Study: Greater weight loss with Atkins-style low-carb diet

A two year Harvard study comparing the low fat American Heart Association diet, a so-called Mediterranean diet, and the low carbohydrate Atkins diet found that the Atkins and Mediterranean diets "are safe and effective options to traditional dieting."

The Atkins dieters—who consumed generous amounts of saturated fat but avoided bread and pasta—saw steeper increases in their HDL, or good cholesterol, than people on either the Mediterranean or low-fat diets, according to results published in the *New England Journal of Medicine*.

The study, funded in part by the Dr. Robert C. and Veronica Atkins Foundation, was the latest to demonstrate the benefits of diets high in fat, protein and cholesterol, which have long been demonized.

"It is time to reconsider the low-fat diet as the first choice for weight loss and for cardiovascular health," said study author Dr. Meir Stampfer of Harvard Medical School. "It is not the best."

— *Sally Squires*, Washington Post, *July 17, 2008*

"Everybody has a story of a neighbor or co-worker who worked out everyday and was nonetheless felled by a heart attack."
— *Stephen L. DeFelice, M.D.*

And don't exercise to death!

The standard medical advice, "exercise and eat a low-fat diet" can be dangerous if you have undiagnosed heart disease. While both mental and physical exercise can enhance and extend life, extreme exercise together with nutritional deficiency may kill you!

Heart pounding exercise can enlarge, stress, and even stop the heart. Like any muscle, the heart benefits from exercise as long as it's not worked beyond its capacity. As William Campbell Douglass, M.D. points out, "Any kind of aerobic exercise, if done more than moderately, can induce atherosclerosis and consequent heart disease."[17]

"The leading cause of exercise-related deaths even in well-trained athletes is coronary heart disease," says Dr Douglass. "Severe coronary atherosclerosis is the most common cause of death in marathon runners…. A compelling argument can be made that over-exercising can cause atherosclerosis and coronary heart disease."[15]

According to Dr. Campbell Douglass, extreme exercise produces a lot of free radicals. "It's not uncommon for highly conditioned athletes and marathon runners to be plagued with colds and infection."[14]

Even though moderate daily exercise is a good idea, it won't result in permanent fat loss. As Taubes writes in *Good Calories Bad Calories*, "Expending more energy than we consume does not lead to long-term weight loss; it leads to hunger." You can work up a big appetite exercising — and then you eat more food.

According to the 2005 federal guidelines, "To help manage body weight and prevent gradual, unhealthy body weight gain in adulthood:"

> "Engage in approximately 60 minutes of moderate-to-vigorous-intensity exercise on most days of the week while not exceeding caloric intake requirements."

Or, "To sustain weight loss in adulthood:"

> "Participate in at least 60 to 90 minutes of daily moderate-intensity exercise while not exceeding caloric intake requirements."

In the real world, let's say a dental assistant works four 10 hour days a week. After 10 hours on her feet, should she go exercise for 60 to 90 minutes? What about the time it takes to do laundry, clean the house, mow the lawn, and prepare meals? Should she eat standing at the kitchen sink? If she has children or older parents to care for, when does she get any rest?

Common sense should tell us that working an 8 or 10 hour day, gardening, shopping, hobbies and any activity that gets us off the coach counts as exercise too. Most of us should aim for 15 to 30 minutes of mild-to-moderate daily exercise. If more demanding exercise interests you, get into it gradually as you improve your nutrition and tone your body.

Also — and most simply — good breathing practices will improve circulation:

> "When you relax, the flow of blood throughout your blood vessels, down to the smallest capillary, is automatically increased without any extra work by the heart."[21]

If your blood pressure or weight is creeping up: Walk, swim, garden, shop on your feet, play cards with friends, go to church, meditate, practice deep breathing, emphasize high quality animal protein and natural fat — and restrict your carbohydrates to 72 grams or less per day.

And quit listening to the experts!

More to Explore...

Recommended fat-loss books, Atkins-style.

• Dr. Robert C. Atkins, *Dr. Atkins Diet Revolution* (New York: David McKay Company, 1972)

> Dr. Atkins' original book, written and published after he had successfully used a high fat carbohydrate-restricted diet on himself and thousands of patients for ten years. This is the classic best-seller describing: "How to lose weight fast eating rich, high-calorie foods."

• Christian B. Allen, PhD and Wolfgang Lutz, MD, *Life Without Bread* (Los Angeles: Keats Publishing, 2000)

> Based on more than forty years of research conducted on over 10,000 patients, *Life Without Bread* unravels the mysteries of nutrition and shows how a low-carbohydrate diet high in healthy fats can reverse — and possibly cure — diabetes, heart disease, and obesity." Provides an easy-to-follow carbohydrate gram counter to help you keep those carbs under 72 grams daily!

• Jan Kwasniewski, *Optimal Nutrition* (Warsaw, Poland: Wydawnictwo, 1999)

> The Polish: "Dr. Atkins." Optimal Nutrition provides the science, rationale, and recipes to help you lose fat permanently without starving or restricting calories. An estimated two or three million people are on the high fat Optimal Diet. Most of these people live in Poland, though news of the diet has spread throughout the world. There are now many optimal high fat eaters in the United States, especially in Chicago.

• Barry Groves, *Natural Health & Weight Loss* (London, UK: Hammersmith Press Ltd., 2007)

> "Barry Groves can claim to be one of Britain's leading exponents of the low-carb/high-fat way of life having lived, researched, lectured and written about this subject for 44 years. In 1982, he took up full-time research into diet and diseases such as obesity, diabetes, heart disease and cancer."

"If the National Cholesterol Education Program was truly concerned about your health, they would be mounting a vigorous nationwide campaign to reduce the American addiction to sugar and refined carbohydrates, which are the real culprits in causing low HDL and oxidized LDL."

— *John R. Lee, M.D.*

CHAPTER 8

Cholesterol is not a medical criminal!

"For the first time, a normal level of a normal, vital body substance is a disease."
— *Malcolm Kendrick, MD, British cardiologist*

What you read in the media about cholesterol is really, really dummied-down. Cholesterol is so vital most cells in the body can make it. Essential for animal life, it is unwise to omit cholesterol from your diet or use drugs to remove it from your blood. It takes a lot of cholesterol to build and maintain a healthy human being, especially a brain!

Cholesterol
$C_{27}H_{45}OH$

We have approximately 100 grams of cholesterol in our bodies; 25 percent in the brain. The highest concentrations are in the connections between nerve cells and in the myelin that protects brain and nervous tissue. Cholesterol is in all cell membranes and is stored in adipose tissue.

Human milk is high in cholesterol because the developing brain and eyes of an infant require large amounts. Cholesterol is the main ingredient in bile, an emulsifier needed for digesting and metabolizing dietary fat. Bile, in turn, protects us by coating and stabilizing slow-moving feces.

Bile is the only way cholesterol leaves the body. Bile is made and excreted at the direction of the liver.

Absorption of dietary cholesterol in the intestines is highly variable, says Professor Michael Gurr, lipid biochemist. He describes how the body's production responds to the amount absorbed in the diet. According to Gurr, "At very high cholesterol intakes, the fraction absorbed decreases, tending to limit absorption."[1]

We have about a tablespoon (10-14 grams) of cholesterol in our blood at any time. When we eat an egg, says lipid biochemist Mary Enig, we absorb about 50 percent or 135 milligrams of cholesterol. Two daily eggs provide no more than 270 mg of absorbed cholesterol — less than 2 percent of blood levels.

> "It is not possible for humans to eat enough cholesterol containing foods every day to supply the amount the body needs," says Dr. Enig. Our liver and other organs have "very active cholesterol-synthesis capability."[2]

Cholesterol starts out in the liver as *acetate*, a common protein-like building block that is recycled to make a variety of things. In turn, cholesterol is a key component of cell membranes throughout the body and a precursor to all steroid and adrenal hormones, including the sex hormones and hormone-like vitamin D.

Technically not a fat, cholesterol is a sterol or high molecular weight alcohol. As "the most important sterol in mammalian tissues," says Professor Gurr, "cholesterol plays a vital role in assuring optimum cell membrane fluidity." (*Sitosterol* and *stigmasterol* are nearly identical sterols that predominate in algae and plants.)[3]

"Different sterols are characteristic of different organisms," says Gurr, principal author of the advanced textbook, *Lipid Biochemistry*. According to Gurr, of all sterols occurring in nature, "Only cholesterol will allow animal membranes to function as required." "Without cholesterol," says Gurr, "our bodies would not function properly and we would die."[4]

Strictly speaking, we do not have "blood cholesterol." Insoluble in water (hydrophobic), cholesterol, fat, and fat soluble vitamins are bundled together into *lipoproteins*, specially designed lipid transport vehicles that can travel in watery blood. From largest to smallest, they are: Chylomicrons, VLDL, LDL and HDL.

According to Gurr, lipid transport systems developed early in evolution. Birds, fishes, amphibians and even roundworms have LDL — they just don't fret about it. Lipoproteins transport cholesterol and fat — either the fat in our diet or the fat made in the liver from dietary sugar or glucose.

Lipoproteins also contain protein, called *apolipoprotein* (apo), which serves as the structural backbone and identifies the lipoprotein to cell receptors throughout the body. As lipoproteins travel in the blood, hungry cells send out the enzyme lipase to snatch up the fat, cholesterol, and fat soluble vitamins.

As an example, when we eat a fatty meal, say two eggs and a lamb chop, the fat and protein begin to separate in the stomach. In the gut, the fat is absorbed into the wall (the enterocyte), broken down into molecules, and then reassembled into a chylomicron, the largest lipoprotein, identified as apoB48 for gut-assembled dietary fat.

Chylomicrons are released into the bloodstream via the lymph and travel until they give up their fatty bounty, shrink, and disappear. Within two or three hours after a fatty meal, chylomicrons — apoB48's — are cleared from the circulation.

(When you fast 12 hours for a "cholesterol check," there is little or no trace of gut-assembled dietary fat circulating in your blood.)

Eat a high carb meal, say two servings of *Kellogg's Raisin Bran* and skim milk, and the metabolism responds in a very different way. Glucose is sent directly into the blood (fructose has to be metabolized in the liver). While this glucose may be used as short term fuel (energy), in well fed people — that's most of us — after a short delay, the liver starts converting excess carbohydrate into the body-made-fat called triglyceride.

The liver bundles this liver-made-fat with cholesterol and protein and sends it out into the bloodstream as very low density lipoprotein (VLDL), identified as apoB100. The second largest lipoprotein, VLDL is the principal hauler of liver-made-fat. VLDL production in the liver is very complex and can go on for several hours after a meal.

The more carbohydrates you eat, the more VLDL is required to transport the liver-made-fat out to the body. As VLDL circulates unloading its load of triglycerides over many hours, it shrinks and morphs into low density lipoprotein (LDL), also identified as apoB100.

VLDL and LDL are a continuum. As VLDL gives up its triglycerides, its function changes and it becomes LDL — delivering mostly cholesterol. Demonized as "bad cholesterol," LDL is not "bad" and its not cholesterol! LDL is the metabolic residue of VLDL; the main carrier of cholesterol to the body.

Triglyceride, technically *triacyglycerol*, is the most common way fat is structured in food and in our bodies. Tri = three (3) fatty acids; glycerol is the backbone. A common triglyceride is three fatty acids "esterified" to glycerol, but in blood work (or a lipid panel), "triglyceride" has a different meaning.

In a lipid panel, triglyceride (TG) is a measure of how much liver-made-fat (apoB100) is circulating in the blood after you fast for 12 hours. In this use of the word, elevated triglycerides (over 100) are a predictive risk factor for heart disease.

Regardless of how much liver-made VLDL is sent out into the circulation, the metabolic system tightly controls its offspring LDL by pulling it out of the blood and recycling it. Homeostatic regulation is the rule with LDL, but VLDL levels depend largely on how much carbohydrate you are eating.

Lipoprotein	Relative Size	Protein Marker	Source	Function
Chylomicrons	bus	ApoB48	Gut	transports dietary fat
VLDL	van	ApoB100	Liver	transports liver-made fat
LDL	car	ApoB100	VLDL	transports cholesterol
HDL	motorcycle	various	Liver	cholesterol mop

The smallest and most numerous lipoprotein, high density lipoprotein (HDL) is secreted separately by the liver and acts as a recycler or cholesterol mop. If the chylomicron is the size of a Greyhound bus, VLDL a van, LDL a compact car, HDL is a fleet of motorcycles hauling cholesterol back to the liver.

Because higher HDL is associated with protection from heart disease, HDL is the most important lipoprotein to test for. Men want HDL over 60; women over 70. HDL and triglycerides have a teeter-totter relationship. As your body is forced to make VLDL to transport triglycerides, an HDL molecule must give up its proteins and disappear.[5]

A 1:1 ratio of triglycerides to HDL — as an example, 90:90 — is protective. A ratio greater than 2:1 alerts you to possible early stages of vascular damage. A 4:1 ratio of triglycerides to HDL — say 150:35 — is the most predictive risk factor for heart disease.

When you have elevated triglycerides and low HDL, your metabolism will result in thicker, clot-prone blood and slow, unrelenting plaque development. *(See Appendix 1, Lipid Panel, to review all heart disease risk factors.)*

As Atkins wrote:

> "The lower you bring down your triglycerides, the less chance you'll have of getting cardiovascular disease. This applies more to women than men; one study estimated that 75 percent of all heart attacks that women get are associated with elevated triglycerides."[6]

High carbohydrate diets are associated with elevated triglycerides and low HDL. Elevated triglycerides are a direct consequence of eating too much carbohydrate. And, as Atkins pointed out, women with elevated triglycerides have a 70 percent higher risk of breast cancer than women with triglycerides below 100.[7]

Heart disease can occur when LDL levels are low, average, or high; but elevated triglycerides, made in the liver from excess carbohydrates, is the most predictive risk factor for coronary heart disease. Also, the higher your triglycerides, the more likely your large fluffy LDL will become a small, dense dangerous particle.

Beyond the scope of this book, there are lipoprotein subfractions. As an example, there is not just one type of LDL or HDL. For this discussion, however, if your triglycerides are elevated, your LDL — regardless of blood level — will more likely be the small, dense variety (subclass B) associated with heart disease.

Obsessed with cholesterol-lowering, most doctors overlook "high normal" blood sugar and elevated triglycerides. According to Dr. Atkins, triglycerides above 100 mg/dl increase your risk of heart attack in a linear manner — the higher the number the greater the risk. Most doctors call triglycerides as high as 150 mg/dl "normal," but then use harsh statin drugs to force "normal" LDL down to less healthy levels.

Don't let them scare you. Total cholesterol is measured in milligrams (mg) per deciliter (dl). A milligram = 1/1000 of a gram, a tiny measure. A deciliter of blood is about 3.4 ounces. In non-diabetic adults over age 50, 180 to 350 mg/dl is a healthy range of blood cholesterol in 3.4 ounces of blood. Fluctuations of "blood cholesterol" due to stress, weather and seasonal changes are also perfectly normal.

The experts are wrong! The American Heart Association fat-phobic, high carbohydrate diet depresses HDL, promotes elevated triglycerides, and is the underling common denominator of obesity, diabetes, and most heart disease. The solution: A traditional American high fat diet.

Dr. Atkins — we love you — you were right all along.

LDL does not predict cardiovascular disease

Dr. Annelies W.E. Weverling-Rijnsburger, from Leiden University in the Netherlands, measured cholesterol levels in 561 subjects who had recently reached age 85. The subjects were then followed for 4 years. During the study period, 152 subjects died and cardiovascular disease was the leading cause of death.

LDL levels were not associated with the risk of death from cardiovascular disease. In contrast, low levels of HDL were associated with mortality. Subjects with HDL below 40 mg/dL were twice as likely to die from stroke or heart disease as participants with HDL levels above 46 mg/dL.

Low levels of both HDL and LDL more than doubled the risk of death from infection. High total cholesterol was associated with a significant reduced risk of death from infection. The authors concluded: "It may be argued that increasing HDL cholesterol levels is more advantageous than lowering total cholesterol levels among old people.

High fat diets — especially saturated fat — are associated with high levels of protective HDL, the so-called good cholesterol. High carb diets — especially sugars and starches — are associated with elevated triglycerides — a dangerous risk factor for heart disease. What are you going to eat for breakfast?

"Watch out for cholesterol that's too low. Anyone with cholesterol under 160 mg/dl has double the risk of brain hemorrhage and an increased risk of leukemia plus cancers of the liver, lung, and pancreas. There's also an increased risk of cirrhosis."

— *Sherry A. Rogers, M.D., author of a new 400 page book,*
The Cholesterol Hoax. Available online at
www.prestigepublishing.com

More to Explore...

Recommended books about cholesterol written by medical doctors between 1973–2007.

- *The Cholesterol Controversy* by Edward R. Pinckney, MD and Cathy Pinckney, (Los Angeles: Sherbourne Press, 1973).

  "There is no scientific evidence to show that high blood cholesterol is the cause of heart disease or that lowering cholesterol – if such a thing is possible – will prevent heart troubles of any kind."

- *The Cholesterol Conspiracy* by Russell L. Smith, PhD, and Edward R Pinckney, MD, (St Louis, Missouri: Warren H. Green, Inc, 1991)

  "Saturated fat and cholesterol in the diet are not the cause of coronary heart disease. That myth is the greatest scientific deception of this century, perhaps of any century."

- *The Cholesterol Myths* by Uffe Ravnskov, MD, PhD (Washington, DC: New Trends Publishing, 2000)

  "A Swedish medical doctor exposes the fallacy that saturated fat and cholesterol cause heart disease."

- *The Great Cholesterol Con* by Malcolm Kendrick, MD, (London, England: John Blake Publishing, 2007)

  "This well documented (and entertaining) book by an English cardiologist confirms the nagging fear that the current cholesterol obsession is utterly misguided."

CHAPTER 9

Lipids for Smart People

"Dietary fat, whether saturated or not, is not a cause of obesity, heart disease or any other chronic disease of civilization."
— *Gary Taubes, author,* Good Calories, Bad Calories

Saturated — King of fats

Caterpillar-like, fatty acids are chains of carbon surrounded by hydrogen. (See illustration below). Carbons join into chains by sharing electrons. When one pair of electrons is shared (**C–C**), a single bond is formed. Fats containing single bonds are called *saturated fats*.

4 Carbon (4C) saturated fat containing single bonds
H H H H **C–C–C–C** All carbons are satisfied **H H H H** (filled) w/hydrogen

"Saturated" means stable — nothing else. The carbons are saturated — satisfied — with hydrogen. Highly saturated coconut oil can sit on your kitchen countertop un-refrigerated for months. With no double bonds, saturated fats are heat stable. Used for centuries, beef fat (tallow) is the right choice for high temperature cooking and frying.

Except water, our cells need fat more than anything else. Cell membranes have two layers of fat called *bilayers*. If cells are tiny houses, *organelles* within cells are the rooms in the house. These rooms or organelles also have fatty bilayers. Saturated fats make up 50 percent or more of the fat in organelle and membrane bilayers.

Unsaturated fat = chemical instability

A double bond is formed when two pairs of electrons are shared (**C=C**). Where there is a double bond, the adjacent carbons are missing hydrogen (**H**). Double bonds (**C=C**) + missing hydrogen (**H**) = chemical instability. Fats with one or more double bonds are chemically unstable and are called unsaturated fat.

Unsaturated fat: One or more double bonds
H H H H
Double bond   **C–C=C–C**   Missing hydrogen
H H H H

An unsaturated fat with one double bond is one (1) or monoun-saturated. Monounsaturated fats are a good choice for moderate heat cooking and frying. Eighteen carbon (18C) oleic acid is the most common monounsaturate, found abundantly in olive oil (and in chicken fat and

Monounsaturated 18 carbon (18C) oleic acid	
18C	**H H H H H H H H H H H H H H H H H H**
Oleic acid	**C–C–C–C–C–C–C–C–C=C–C–C–C–C–C–C–C–C**
One double bond	**H H H H H H H H H H H H H H H H H H**

lard).

Polyunsaturated fats have two or more double bonds and are very (poly) unstable. Reactive to heat, light, and oxygen, commercial polyun-saturates are derived from their source with heat, light, and oxygen — and often chemical solvents like hexane. Cooking with them generates more heat, light, and oxygen.

Polyunsaturated fat: 2 or more double bonds	
18C *Linoleic acid* Two double bonds	H H H H H H H H H H H H H H H H H H C–C–C–C–C–C–C–C–C=C–C–C=C–C–C–C–C–C H H H H H H H H H H H H H H H

Classified "good" by federal nutrition authorities, polyunsaturated corn, safflower, soybean, and sunflower oils have no place in your kitchen. Once ingested, these highly processed inherently unstable vegetable fats are incorporated into our membranes where they promote injury and inflammation. (See Unsafe *At Any Meal*, page 92 of this chapter).

Our bodies are made of fat and protein. If we eat too much heat-damaged vegetable fat, we are, in Atkins' words, "cooking ourselves from the inside." When unsaturated fat is hydrogenated — to make fast food and highly processed packaged foods — the not-found-in-nature trans fatty acids are formed.

Trans Fatty Acids (TFAs)

Trans fatty acids have been in margarine and vegetable shortening since *Crisco* vegetable shortening was introduced in 1912. Trans fats have been the fat of mass destruction for decades in commercial baked foods and in virtually all highly processed foods — like fast food French fries and chicken *McNuggets*.

Trans fatty acids (TFAs) are found in unsaturated fats that have been industrially hydrogenated — a high pressure, high temperature process that causes the hydrogen atoms to "jump" across at the double bond. These chemical changes give the fat very long shelf life and make it more

Trans **bond** (**H** opposite each other)	*Cis* **bond** (**H** same side of double bond)
H H C=C H H	H H C=C H H

functional for food processing.

The natural cis bond (above, right) has hydrogen on the same side of the double bond. Our enzyme systems are designed to deal with the cis-configuration. The trans bond on the left was created by industrial hydrogenation. Once ingested, these trans fatty acids create havoc in our membranes.

These are the fats recommended by the American Heart Association in their 1956 television fundraiser and in their 1961 first official "low fat" diet. These are the same fats recommended by the young, naïve staffers in Senator McGovern's 1977 Dietary Goals for the U.S. and in all nutrition guidelines between 1980 and 2000.

> "Everyone in health food stores looks pale. Everybody at the Carnegie Deli looks healthy."
>
> — *Jackie Mason, comedian*

Yahoo! Food's "The Ultimate Guide to Good and Bad Fats"

Like the dummied-down information about cholesterol, the misinformation about saturated fat is promoting endless confusion about what to eat. As a recent example, *Yahoo!* Food's "The Ultimate Guide to Good and Bad Fats," asserts:

> "Saturated fats are mainly trouble because they raise blood cholesterol to artery-clogging levels."[1]

Yahoo! advises us to "skimp or skip" on "Lousy Saturated Fats," including: Red meat, chicken skin, butter and lard. But any lipid biochemist will tell you that fat in food is always a complex mixture of different fatty acids — saturated and unsaturated:

The most saturated fats (like coconut) contain mono- and polyunsaturates, and the most polyunsaturated fats (like flaxseed) contain saturated and monounsaturated fat.

Beef fat is 45 percent unsaturated
Chicken skin is 70 percent unsaturated
Butter is 30 percent unsaturated
Lard is 60 percent unsaturated

The following chart illustrates how full fat milk and butter — the most complex of all food fats — is not "artery-clogging-saturated fat." Full fat milk and butter contain 12 different fatty acids, including 8 different saturated fats with 8 different chain lengths. (Please note that milk fat is also more than 30 percent unsaturated fat.)

Percent	Type/Acid	Chain length	# double bonds
Composition of Milk Fat and Butter			
4	butyric	4	0 = saturated
2	caproic	6	0
1	caprylic	8	0
2	capric	10	0
3	lauric	12	0
12	myristic	14	0
26	palmitic	16	0
12	stearic	18	0
2	palmitoleic	16	1 = monounsaturated
28	oleic	18	1
3	linoleic	18	2 = polyunsaturated
<1	alpha linolenic	18	3 = polyunsaturated

2-3 percent odd chain fatty acids

As an example, butter is 26 percent *palmitic acid*, the most common saturated fat found in plants, animals, and microorganisms (see above). As a stem-fatty acid, palmitic acid is used by our bodies to make other fatty acids and is the major surfactant protecting human lungs:

> 68 percent of the fat covering our lungs is saturated palmitic acid, found abundantly in palm oil, lard, chicken skin, and butter.

Unlike cholesterol, found only in animal membranes, we share fats with plants, animals, and microorganisms. To continue the example of palmitic acid: olive oil and peanut oils are 12 to 14 percent palmitic; chicken fat, and lard (from a pig) are 25 to 26 palmitic; tropical palm oil — where the name comes from — is 45 percent palmitic acid.

Your body can't tell the difference between palmitic acid in palm oil and palmitic acid in lard or chicken skin. They are identical. According to lipid biochemist Mary Enig, Ph.D:

> "Basic fatty acids are the same molecules whether they come from plants or animals (including people)."[2]

Not only is fat in food a complex mixture of saturated and unsaturated fats; but, equally important, the metabolism of saturated fat varies widely. As an example, stearic acid, an 18 carbon saturated fat found in beef, lamb, butter, and chocolate, raises protective HDL cholesterol and helps reduce the "bad" elevated triglycerides associated with risk of heart disease.

As lipid biochemist Michael Gurr points out:

> "It is clear that suggestions that saturated fatty acids differed in their cholesterol — raising capacities were already apparent in the 1950s and certainly in the 1960s" — when the American Heart Association condemned all saturated fats as "bad."

In his textbook, *Lipid Biochemistry*, Professor Gurr lists fifteen (15) naturally occurring saturated fats with chain lengths ranging from 2 to 28 carbons. "Chain length has a profound effect on the capacity of saturated fatty acids to raise plasma total cholesterol," says Gurr — and *only saturated fats* with chain lengths of 12, 14, and 16 have that "potential."

The following chart of eight (8) common saturated fats illustrates how sweeping statements about "saturated fats raising cholesterol" are not useful. Please note both the variety of chain lengths in the different saturates and their differing relative potential to raise cholesterol.

No. of Carbons	Common Name	Potential To Raise LDL	Occurrence in food
The Eight Most Common Saturated Fats			
4	Butyric	no	In milk fat of ruminants
6	Caproic	no	Milk fat
8	Caprylic	no	Very minor component/most animal & plant fats Major component/many milk and some seed fats
10	Capric	no	Widespread as a minor component; major component of many milk and some seed fats
12	Lauric	yes	Widely distributed/major component of palm kernel/coconut oil/human breast milk
14	Myristic	yes	Widespread, occasionally found as a major component
16	Palmitic	yes	The most common saturated fatty acid found in animals, plants and microorganisms
18	Stearic	no	Major component in animals; minor constituent in plants; major constituent in cocoa butter

In summary, according to Gurr:

"Dietary saturated fatty acid - plasma lipid interrelationships have been grossly oversimplified. Old simplistic statements, such as "saturated fats raise plasma cholesterol, need to be reappraised…"[3]

Lipid metabolism is very complex: "The extent to which these fatty acids raise cholesterol is dependent on the concentration of linoleic acid in the dietary mix [omega 6 polyunsaturated fat] and possibly interactions with other dietary components."[4]

"A recent study clearly shows that if dietary fat composition is maintained constant, dietary fat level has little or no influence on the concentration of cholesterol in the blood."

And, finally: "of the various dietary factors that affect plasma cholesterol, cholesterol in food plays a minor role..."[5]

We've been mislead about saturated fat and cholesterol for 40 years! And even if a saturated fat like palmitic acid has the potential to raise blood cholesterol — if you're over 50 — statistically speaking — you'll live longer!

The bottom line:

Saturated fat is the fall guy for the huge profits generated for five decades by the really big oil companies: those that make vegetable oil.

Besides, the hype about fat affecting cholesterol is overblown!

Unlike blood sugar, which has a narrow optimum range of 85 to 95, blood cholesterol has a wide "normal" range of 180 to 350 mg/dl. While excess sugar turns to fat, cholesterol — in response to stress, weather and other factors — will migrate between blood and tissue to satisfy the body's complex needs.

The folks at Yahoo! — like most of us — have been sold a bill of goods about "Good and Bad fats." When choosing cooking fats, just remember the best options for baking and cooking are the traditional, more stable saturated and monounsaturated fats found in animal tallow, butter, chicken, lard, olive, coconut and palm oils — the safe, proven fats humans have eaten for centuries!

As we shall learn in the final sections of this chapter, highly processed vegetable fats — whether hydrogenated (trans fat) or not — are the *Fats of Mass Destruction*. Both excess linoleic acid (omega 6) and excess heat-damaged linoleic acid damage cell membranes and cause inflammatory fires throughout the body.

Linoleic acid: Unsafe at any meal

Dr. Paul Beaumont, Ophthalmologist with the Macular Degeneration Foundation, has seen a tenfold increase in macular degeneration in the last 30 years. "I've seen an exponential rise from the early 1970s through the 1990s," says Dr. Beaumont.[6]

"I don't think there's any doubt we have an epidemic."

Today, macular degeneration has overtaken diabetes as the leading cause of vision loss in the U.S. and affects more than 10 million Americans. Macular degeneration is caused by the deterioration of the central portion of the retina, called the macula. The macula controls our ability to read, drive a car, and recognize faces and colors.

According to Bruce Fife, N.D., "Over the past few years, several studies have linked polyunsaturated vegetable oils with macular degeneration." According to Fife, "If your diet includes soybean, corn and other highly processed vegetable oils, you may be at high risk for developing age-related macular degeneration."[7]

The research cited by Fife shows that "people who eat polyunsaturated vegetable oils get macular degeneration twice as commonly as those who don't." According to Fife, saturated fat has the lowest risk; the higher the degree of unsaturation, the greater the risk.[8]

The oils you have to watch out for are soybean, safflower, corn and other polyunsaturated fats, including margarine and partially hydrogenated vegetable oils. Olive oil is the safest vegetable fat to cook with because it contains a higher percentage of stable saturated and monounsaturated fat.

As we have learned, fats and oils are not reserved for energy. They are incorporated into our cell membranes, and — once ingested — chemically unstable polyunsaturated vegetable oils are highly susceptible to lipid peroxidation, the chemical process that causes fats to spew out free radicals!

Oxidized vegetable fats interfere with normal cell function, leading to many illnesses, including macular degeneration. Rancid oils create destructive free radicals. Free radicals rip into other molecules, causing irreversible damage to cells. When this happens in the retina, you may go blind.

Among dietary fats, stable coconut oil (90 percent saturated) and beef tallow (60 percent saturated) are two of the traditional fats we should be using in the kitchen. Before the Center for Science in the Public Interest (CSPI) launched its *Anti-Saturated Fat Attack* — financed in part by vegetable oil lobbyists — food producers, restaurants, and fast food enterprises were using safe, stable animal tallows and the healthy tropical saturates.

4-hydroxy-trans-2-nonenal (HNE)

To make these oils even worse, a toxin called 4-hydroxy-trans-2-nonenal (HNE) forms in especially high amounts in vegetable oils that contain linoleic acid, which include canola, corn, soybean and sunflower oils.[9] The compound does not arise in the saturated fats found in coconut oil, beef tallow, or lard.

"It's a very toxic compound," states A.Saari Csallany, a professor of food chemistry and nutritional biochemistry at the University of Minnesota. According to Csallany, numerous studies have linked vegetable oil consumption to increased risk for cardiovascular disease, stroke, Parkinson's, Alzheimer's, Huntington's disease, liver ailments, and cancer.[10]

"This toxic compound — HNE — has been shown to incorporate into food during frying and is readily absorbed from the diet," says Csallany. "It is capable of reacting with amino acids, DNA, and other biomolecules."

> "It reacts with various kinds of amino groups — proteins, DNA, RNA, affecting basic cellular processes."[11]

Vegetable-based polyunsaturated fats are inherently unstable, especially at higher cooking temperatures. All vegetable oils contain linoleic acid. It is the linoleic acid in these oils that converts to HNE during cooking. The more linoleic acid, the more HNE formed during cooking.

If that's not enough, research done at Stockholm University shows that baking or frying carbohydrate-rich foods like potatoes and grains forms *acrylamide*, a probable human carcinogen. The Swedish scientists found that a bag of potato chips could contain up to 500 times more acrylamide than the maximum levels allowed in drinking water by the World Health Organization.[12]

According to the free online encyclopedia, *Wikipedia*:

> "Acrylamide was accidentally discovered in foods in April 2002 by scientists in Sweden when they found large amounts of the chemical in starchy foods, such as potato chips, French fries and bread that had been heated..."[13]

New York City bans trans fat — but the replacement — Interesterified fat — raises blood sugar in humans

In 2005, New York was the first city to outlaw the use of partially hydrogenated trans fat in restaurants, a ban now being considered in other cities across the U.S. But the favored substitute is no better — and may be worse!

Research published in Nutrition and Metabolism (2007, 4:3) shows that *interesterification*, the new favored method of modifying fat in commercial products, raises blood sugar and depresses insulin response in humans — common precursors to diabetes.[14]

This means companies are swapping out very bad *trans* for a new dangerous fat. The *Nutrition and Metabolism* study shows that interesterification, which unnaturally rearranges the fatty acids in the triglycerides, can alter metabolism in humans.

In the study, protective HDL cholesterol dropped slightly with both the trans fat and interesterified blends, but the real problem concerned blood glucose and insulin levels:

> "Insulin levels dropped 10 percent on the partially hydrogenated soybean oil but dropped more than twice as much on the interesterified diet — causing blood sugar to rise by an alarming 20 percent."[15]

While the word is finally out on the dangers of trans fat, most New Yorkers and other Americans think they are safe eating the new yummy "trans-free" oils. Guess again.

According to lipid biochemist Dr. Mary Enig, the New York City uproar over trans fat provided an ideal opportunity to bring back our traditional more stable saturated fats, but "the vegetable oil industry has been working overtime behind the scenes to make sure that doesn't happen."

According to Dr. Enig:

> "They have hired PR firms to get articles published in journals and popular media warning the public about the evils of saturated fats."[16]

An impartial review of the evidence more than suggests that our current intake of highly processed vegetable oils is damaging our health. In 1910, Americans consumed less than one pound of vegetable oil per year. Today, that figure is 75 pounds. No human — including us nutritionally hapless Americans — were designed to eat so much highly processed vegetable fat.

We are getting too much omega 6 — and too much damaged omega 6 — and not enough essential omega 3, found in wild game, organ meat (liver), lamb, grass fed beef, free range eggs, flaxseed, and walnuts. An excess of omega 6 constricts blood vessels, raises blood pressure, creates life-threatening arrhythmia, and provokes inflammation in the blood vessels.

Both the clear harm of excess vegetable oil and the continuing decades-old shenanigans of the vegetable oil industry remain largely unknown to the U.S. public. Buyer beware! The best cooking fats are those with the least amount of linoleic acid, trans fat, and interesterified fat.

It's time to limit, restrict, or boycott:
- Any margarine or vegetable shortening
- Polyunsaturated cooking oils in clear plastic bottles
- Hydrogenated or partially hydrogenated vegetable oil
- Trans-fatty acids
- Interesterified vegetable fat
- Heat-damaged pasteurized, homogenized milk
- Low fat or skim milk with synthetic vitamin D added
- Egg-Beaters
- Agribusiness' widespread use of antibiotic drugs
- Feedlot, confined farm animals
- Olestra fake fat and all fat substitutes.
- Official government low-fat diets

"Butter added to vegetables and spread on bread, and cream added to soups and sauces, ensures proper assimilation of the minerals and water-soluble vitamins in vegetables, grains, and meat."
— *Sally Fallon,* Nourishing Traditions

"There is nothing unsafe about butter; quite the opposite, butter contains healthful components that are not found in anything else (other than real cream)."
— *Mary Enig,* Know Your Fats

More to Explore

The information in this chapter was consolidated largely from the research and writings of biochemists Mary G. Enig and Michael I. Gurr. To learn more about lipid nutrition and kitchen fats and oils, consult:

• *Know Your Fats* by Mary G. Enig, Ph.D. Written for lay people, *Know Your Fats* offers a "complete primer for understanding the nutrition of fats, oils, and cholesterol." Dr. Enig is a nutritionist, biochemist of international renown, and Vice President of the Weston A. Price Foundation. She has headed a number of studies on the content and effects of trans fatty acids in America and Israel and has successfully challenged government assertions that dietary animal fat causes cancer and heart disease.

• *Lipids In Nutrition: A Reappraisal* by Michael I. Gurr, PhD., is a compilation of 60 articles on lipid nutrition written by Professor Gurr and published in the journal *Lipid Technology* between 1989-98. "There is a growing awareness that some of the conclusions of the early nutrition experiments were not of the best design, that conclusions sometimes went beyond the experimental evidence, that the lipid hypothesis for cardiovascular disease, for example, is far from the whole story, and that early conclusions about cholesterol and saturated fat need to be reconsidered."

• *Lipid Biochemistry, 5th Edition,* by professors Michael I. Gurr, John L. Harwood, and Keith N. Frayn. This advanced textbook is written for upper level students of biochemistry, biology, nutrition, and food science. In particular, *Lipid Biochemistry* is an invaluable, authoritative resource for understanding: fatty acid metabolism, lipid transport, lipids in cellular structures, and the metabolism of structural lipids. Find online at www.blackwell-science.com.

• *The Good Fat Cookbook* by Fran McCullough. "The Good Fat Cookbook provides even more evidence that the foods we love to eat — butter, chocolate, coconut, whole milk and cream, nuts avocados, cold-water fish and red meat, olive oil, bacon and eggs — are actually good for us."

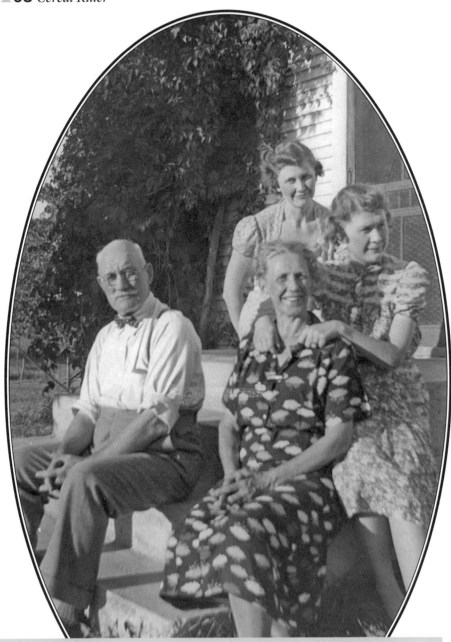

"It's time to put pigs back on the farm and lard back in the kitchen"

— *Alan L. Watson*

CHAPTER 10

Praise the Lard

"The stage might be set at last for the comeback of the great misunderstood fat: lard."
— *Corby Kummer, Senior Editor,* Atlantic Monthly

Yes, lard — the creamy white fat of pigs. We're talking about the fat from outdoor-living, properly-raised healthy animals. Like other foods, lard can be a healthy choice or best avoided. Most supermarket lard has been partially hydrogenated, contains trans fat, and is rendered from confined, indoor animals.

Traditionally-rendered lard from outdoor pigs has been a primary cooking fat for centuries in China, Japan, South America, parts of Europe and in the United States until the 1920s. In 1910, lard represented 70 percent of the edible fat market in the U.S., but lard consumption declined to less than 2 pounds per capita by the year 2000.

Leaf lard, considered the finest quality, comes from the fatty deposit around the kidneys. Back fat, a hard layer between the flesh and the skin, is also highly regarded. The fat left in the pan after frying bacon is lard (with a little protein). Despite centuries of safe use, the American Heart Association has demonized lard as an "artery clogging saturated fat."

But lard is more unsaturated (60 percent) than saturated (40 percent). Depending on the pigs' diet, lard is dominantly monounsaturated oleic acid with a fatty composition not unlike olive oil. Like all food fats, lard is a complex mixture, including saturated (40 percent), monounsaturated (50 percent), and polyunsaturated (10 percent) fat.

In *The Good Fat Cookbook*, author and chef Fran McCullough writes:

> "Of the part of pork that is saturated fat (about 40 percent), a third of that is the very good stearic acid, which has a beneficial effect on cholesterol and relaxes blood vessels."[1]

In a recent *NY Times* editorial, Corby Kummer, senior editor at *Atlantic Monthly*, had only praise for lard. "Lard makes the lightest and tastiest fried chicken: Buttermilk, secret spices and ancient cast iron skillets are all well and good, but the key to fried chicken greatness is lard."[2]

Pork has been used since man first learned to grow crops and domesticate animals. Once salting and smoking were discovered as methods of preservation, pork became a valuable food for the lean winter months. Pork is the best food source of vitamin B1, (thiamine), important for carbohydrate metabolism and appetite control.

In many regions where pigs thrive, fattening them became part of family life, and the butchering of pigs coincided with the fall harvest. Pork and its fat became associated with the English and American holidays: Succulent Christmas ham and potatoes roasted in lard. Smart holiday bakers will tell you there is no substitute for lard when making pastries and pie crust.

According to food scientist Harold McGee, lard — like other lipids — forms crystals just below the melting point. Lard is better suited for pastries because "It forms large crystals that impart a noticeably grainy texture to the dough — which produces the sought after flakiness."[4]

Traditional Hungarian chefs use lard because the high smoke point (400 degrees) allows the paprika to release a higher percentage of its color and flavors. The best Mexican cuisine is redolent of lard, says Zarela Martinez, chef and owner of the Manhattan restaurant Zarela.

When asked if she cooks with lard, her answer:

> "Yes, yes, I love lard, I use it when I want its flavor, as in refried beans, or the lightness and fluffiness it brings to tamales, or the crispness it gives to pastries and fried *antojitos*, or the way it melds the flavors of the countless ingredients in moles."[3]

In his book *Hog Heaven*, Lyall Watson comments on the "indispensable" role lard played in opening up the American West:

> "Mixed with petroleum it produced grease and combined with lye it made soap. It protected meat from spoilage, preserved a whole range of foods by sealing them from the air — and catered to everyone's health and pleasure until 20th century dieticians spoiled the fun."[5]

Lard lowdown

One piece of "Hog Heaven" today is the north side of Chicago where 2,000 Polish Americans — and 2 million people worldwide — are following the *Optimal Diet*, a high fat eating plan developed decades ago by Polish physician, Jan Kwasniewski, MD. While working in a Polish military sanitarium, Dr. Kwasniewski discovered that his sick patients were simply suffering from "bad nutrition."

After a couple decades refining his theory, in 1990, Kwasniewski published *Optimal Nutrition* (in Polish), outlining an eating plan that calls for consuming three grams of fat for each gram of protein and half gram of carbohydrate: Fat: 3, Protein: 1, and carbohydrate: ½. The Optimal Diet calls for eating prodigious amounts of animal fat — preferably lard.[6]

Lech Walesa, eating plenty of fatty pork, eggs, and lard, reportedly lost 44 pounds and reversed type 2 diabetes on the "Polish Atkins diet." Like Atkins, the Optimal Diet restricts grains and sugars and recommends that we eat up to 250 grams of animal fat per day.[7]

According to the *Chicago Tribune*, Dr. Kwasniewski's devotees gather around the Optimal Deli in Portage Park, Illinois, to share success stories. Like the fat in the Optimal Diet there are plenty. Josef Ostrowski, 71, says he's been eating pork meat, liver, blood sausage and lard all his life — he just didn't know it was healthy until he read Dr. Kwasniewski's book.[8]

Chicago Physician Christopher Kubik has been on the diet for 4 years. He lost 25 pounds in six weeks and reached his ideal weight. He is no longer plagued with bladder stones and feels much more energetic eating fried eggs, bacon, and string cheese for breakfast seven days a week.

Kubik, who has degrees in public health and health law, doesn't actively promote the Optimal Diet "because it is not considered a standard of care and the medical community still recommends low-fat diets and it is not something I could support if I were sued." But if patients ask, "I tell them that I am on it and have seen positive results." [for 4 years.][9]

While Kwasniewski and other doctors face harassment and prosecution for recommending healthy traditional fats eaten safely for centuries across the globe, most Americans are deficient in the fat soluble vitamins abundant in these condemned fats, especially vitamin D.

Lard and vitamin D

In *Nutrition and Physical Degeneration*, first published in 1939, Canadian-born dentist Weston A. Price documented how the diets of so called primitive or traditional people contained "at least ten times" more fat soluble vitamins A and D as the standard American diet of his day.

Agreeing with Weston Price, contemporary Canadian researcher Dr. Reinhold Vieth provides convincing evidence that current vitamin D recommendations (200-400 IU) do not come close to the amounts necessary for optimum health. According to Dr. Vieth, the minimum daily requirement of vitamin D from all sources is approximately 4,000 IUs.[10]

Cod liver oil is highest in vitamin D, followed by lard. Without using the foods listed below on a regular basis, it is difficult to obtain 4,000 IUs daily from food. Two teaspoons of cod liver oil (500 IU per teaspoon) plus generous amounts of lard, herring, oysters, sardines, butter, and egg yolk are required.

Food Sources of Vitamin D (for 100 grams or about 3 ½ ounces)[11]

Cod Liver Oil	10,000
Lard (pork fat)	2,800
Pickled Atlantic Herring	680
Steamed Eastern Oysters	542
Steamed/poached Catfish	500
Skinless Sardines	480
Canned/Drained Mackerel	450
Smoked Chinook Salmon	320
Sturgeon Roe	232
Canned/Drained Shrimp	172

Fresh Egg Yolk 148

Butter. 56

From The Miracle of Vitamin D *by Krispin Sullivan, CN*

Like pigs, humans manufacture vitamin D from sunlight. In a complex process, *UV-B* rays must first reach cholesterol in the skin. In most climates, however, it is difficult to obtain enough vitamin D without spending several hours per week at midday in the sun with much of your skin exposed.

Pioneer Americans ate lard — the number one cooking fat until 1940. Lard from naturally-raised pigs provided abundant vitamin D while butter and meat from grass-fed pastured cows was a rich source of vitamin A. In combination, fat soluble A and D from animal fats are the catalysts for mineral absorption required for good health.

According to Krispin Sullivan, it is now well established that vitamin D is required for the absorption of calcium, magnesium, iron and zinc. Vitamin D receptors are found throughout the body, and research since the 1980s documents that optimum levels of vitamin D contribute to a healthy immune system, promote muscle strength, regulate the maturation process, and contribute to hormone production.[12]

During the last ten years, Sullivan and other researchers have documented that vitamin D:

🐖 Protects lipids (fat and cholesterol) from oxidation.

🐖 Promotes the synthesis and release of insulin.

🐖 Guards against cataracts forming in the eyes.

🐖 Protects against Polycystic Ovarian Syndrome.

🐖 Helps prevent auto immune diseases such as M.S., Sjogren's Syndrome, rheumatoid arthritis, and Crohn's disease.

🐖 Protects against osteoporosis in diets that include sufficient calcium, magnesium and trace minerals.

🐖 Supports the production of natural estrogen in men and women.

🐖 Guards against breast, prostate, skin and colon cancer.

Since the 1960s, Americans have not only markedly reduced their consumption of lard and other animal fats, but they have dramatically increased their intake of polyunsaturated oils and hydrogenated fats. Trading animal fats for highly processed vegetable fats has contributed to widespread vitamin D deficiencies.

The absorption and utilization of vitamin D is influenced by the kinds of fats we consume. Excess polyunsaturated and monounsaturated fats from vegetable oils decrease the binding of vitamin D to the D-binding proteins. Saturated fats do not have this effect, nor do the omega 3 fats found abundantly in fatty fish.

Lard Composition			
Percent	Type/Acid	Chain length	# double bonds
1	myristic	14	0
25	palmitic	16	0
12	stearic	18	0
3	palmitoleic	16	1 = monounsaturated
45	oleic	18	1
10	linoleic	18	2 = polyunsaturated
<1	alpha linolenic	18	3 = polyunsaturated

Myristic acid (14C saturated fat) occurs widely in most animal and plant fats. It is used in metabolism involving stabilization of some of the cellular proteins. (Nutmeg butter is a major source at 70-80 percent.)

Palmitic acid (16C saturated fat) is the most common saturated fatty acid in plants, animals, and microorganisms. Palmitic is called the "stem" fatty acid because it is the basic fatty acid made in the body and constitutes 68 percent of human lung surfactant.

Stearic acid (18C saturated fat) is found most abundantly in beef and cocoa butter (35 percent). Stearic acid raises protective HDL and lowers elevated triglycerides.

Palmitoleic acid (16C monounsaturated fat) possesses antimicrobial properties. (At 23 percent, macadamia nuts are highest in palmitoleic acid.)

Oleic acid (18C monounsaturated fat) is found in all animal and vegetable fats. It is made in the human body from stearic acid. Oleic acid is the dominant fat in olive oil.

Linoleic acid (18C polyunsaturated fat) is the basic omega 6 fatty acid with two double bonds.

Alpha linolenic acid is (18C polyunsaturated fat is the basic omega 3 fatty acid with three double bonds.

Going Forward

Based on the evidence cited by a legion of highly respected scientific researchers, it's clear that almost everything we have been lead to believe about weight loss and the nature of a heart-healthy diet is wrong — especially that fat is bad — carbs are good.

With tens of millions acting on this advice, we are witnessing an unprecedented increase in obesity, diabetes, and heart failure. The problem lies with the emphasis on carbohydrates in the federal nutrition guidelines and the recommendation to replace animal fats with highly processed vegetable fats.

If you are pre-diabetic or have pounds to burn, emphasize low glycemic carbohydrates — or don't eat any at all. Remember, carbs are not biological essentials! The liver can convert fat into ketone bodies to fuel the brain and nervous system — and protein (in the diet or muscles) can be converted into glucose and used as a secondary fuel.

Since carbs are not required, why eat them in excess? It's easier than you think to eliminate dry boxed cereals, heat-damaged watery milk, breakfast bars, "grain candy," soft drinks, and highly processed chips and sugary snacks. Optimum blood sugar control means eating no more than 50-72 grams of carbohydrate per day — chosen mostly from the vegetable kingdom.

In *Life Without Bread*, Wolfgang Lutz, MD, suggests eating no more than what he describes as six (6) bread units (BU) of carbohydrate per day — each BU containing 12 grams of utilizable carbohydrate. Lutz has studied low-carbohydrate nutrition for 40 years and recommends a high fat diet to reverse and cure diabetes and heart disease. *(Read about Dr. Lutz's book, Chapter 7, page 75.)*

As in the Atkins diet, any foods that contain no carbohydrate can be eaten freely (high quality meats, cheese, fish, eggs, butter), but carbohydrates should not exceed 72 grams per day. As an example, the following carbohydrate choices provide 72 grams of carbohydrate:

Bread Unit	Selected Food
1 bread unit each =	1 slice of bread
12 grams carbohydrate	2/3 cups of peas
	½ of a medium potato
	1 cup of broccoli
	1 medium apple
	1 cup of whole milk

Above all else, disregard the carbohydrate-emphasized federal nutrition guidelines, calorie-counting, and fear-based eating. If you have fat to lose, change your fuel to fat. Like Atkins' experience in 1963, you may have the surprise of your life. You'll burn the fat you want to lose and regain the vital energy you need to live a full and happy life.

Your daily fare should emphasize high quality animal protein and a variety of natural fats — plant and animal. If you shop the outer isle at the supermarket or buy direct from the farmer or farmer's market, it's hard to go wrong. Since restoring our health depends on optimum levels of the forgotten fat soluble vitamins, we need to support the old fashioned farms and farmers that produce them.

For healthy children and vital adults, we must restore our traditional higher fat whole foods diet into the 2010 revised federal nutrition guidelines. It's time to praise the lard, pass the butter, and bring back the tropical saturated fats — coconut and palm. Instead of skimping on meat and animal foods, it's time to support the old-fashioned farmers who know the value of animals on pasture.

Use butter, olive oil, coconut, palm, or lard for cooking

In *Nourishing Traditions*, Sally Fallon recommends using extra virgin olive oil for cooking and unrefined flax oil for salad dressings. She suggests coconut oil for baking and animal fats such as lard for occasional frying. Finally, she says, use as much good quality butter as you like.

In *Know Your Fats*, Mary Enig recommends coconut oil for popcorn. For baking, she recommends butter, coconut oil, lard, palm oil, and animal tallow (drippings). She also offers her own all-purpose recipe for sautéing and light frying: One-third each coconut oil, sesame oil, and olive oil.

(The coconut oil needs to be warmed to about 80 degrees before mixing.) Teaspoon, tablespoon, and cup measures all work.

"Our choice of fats and oils is of extreme importance," says Fallon. Her recommendation is to avoid all processed foods that contain hydrogenated fats and polyunsaturated oils.

Enig's advice is to "consume optimal amounts of fat-soluble vitamins A, D, E, and K, found in animal fats." She says adults and children should eat at least one whole egg a day. Enig recommends full fat dairy products, especially for children.

> "In 2005, for the first time since 1957, Americans ate more butter than margarine – six-tenths of a pound more per person, to be exact. Okay, so that may not sound like an extraordinary figure, but, boy, does it make me (and my father) happy"
> — *James Oseland, Editor-in-Chief,* Saveur *magazine*

Both Fallon and Enig recommend eating anything made with coconut oil or products made with desiccated or whole coconut such as macaroons or coconut milk. Coconut is the best source of antimicrobial lauric acid.

Finally, both Fallon and Enig emphasize the need to include healthy fats from a wide variety of natural meats, fish, seeds, and vegetables. Do not rely on just one fat or oil exclusively.

Sally Fallon and Dr. Mary Enig are president and vice president respectively of the Weston A. Price Foundation, founded in 1999 to disseminate the research and continue the mission of Dr. Price. The Foundation is dedicated to restoring nutrient-dense foods to the American diet through education, research, and activism. Projects they support include accurate nutrition education, organic and biodynamic farming, pasture-feeding of livestock, and community supported farms.

Two important current goals include promoting unfettered universal access to clean certified raw milk (www.realmilk.com) — and, conversely, working to ban the use of soy formula for infants through their Soy Alert Project. Contact the Foundation by calling 202-333-HEAL or online at www.westonaprice.org.

Federal nutrition revisions are due in 2010

As you finish this book, a lot of behind-the-scenes maneuvering and a new advertising campaign to influence the 2010 revisions are underway. In September, 2008, the corn-syrup industry — including Archer Daniels Midland and Cargill — launched a $20 to $30 million 18-month campaign to argue that their corn sweetener is no worse than white sugar.[13]

More than 10 percent of Americans' daily calories come from high fructose corn syrup, and now the Corn Refiners Association is gearing up to make sure they have "a sweeter image" going into 2010. According to Audrae Erickson, the association's president, the 18-month ad campaign "will target mostly mothers" — and the $30 million will be well spent![14]

It's time for American mothers (and fathers) to rid themselves and their children of all forms of excess sugar — especially high fructose corn syrup — and reign in the lobbyists from the soft drink, sugar, fructose, and cereal industries who are dead set on spending tens of millions to protect their huge profits even at the expense of America's children — and America's future.

More to Explore...
Books that challenge politically correct nutrition.

• Sally Fallon, *Nourishing Traditions* (Washington DC: New Trends Publishing, 1999)

"The Diet Dictocrats don't want you to know that...
—Your body needs old-fashioned animal fats
—New-fangled polyunsaturated oils are bad for you
—Modern whole grain products cause health problems
—Traditional sauces promote digestion and assimilation
—Modern food processing denatures our food
—Ancient methods actually increase nutrients

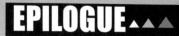

Be careful with whom you trust your heart...

"Yea, though I walk through the valley of the shadow of death, I will fear no evil: for thou art with me; thy rod and thy staff comfort me."

— *Psalm 23*

My mother's parents were dairy farmers in Meadow Township just outside the small northern town of Sebeka, Minnesota. My Finnish grandfather raised work horses and grazed cows, sheep, and hogs on his 160-acre "mixed farm."

My grandmother Emma's many chores included milling grains and baking coarse whole grain bread two or three times a week. My mother helped in the kitchen and made sure the chickens were fed. My mother's older sister and brother worked as field hands.

My grandfather's pigs rooted in the ground (how they get their iron) and lapped up the abundant skimmed milk. The valuable milk fat was delivered to the busy Sebeka Creamery where it was made into delicious butter and then sent by train as far away as New York City.

(In 1936, the farmer-owned Sebeka Cooperative Creamery produced a record 1,818,108 pounds of sweet cream butter from the area's grass-fed cows.)

There was abundance and tragedy. Infant daughter Lila died during the 1918 flu epidemic. Lightning struck and burned down my grandfather's barn, killing his prized work horses. Times were tough in the 30s, but the farm prospered and the family remembered "eating well."

My mother graduated from high school in 1937 and moved to Portland, Oregon to work as a nanny for "a wealthy Jewish family." (Go West young woman, go West!) Bombs falling on Pearl Harbor, December 7, 1941, brought her right back home to northern Minnesota.

My mother met my father on a blind date in 1940s wartime Minneapolis. My father was on leave from the army, and it was love at first sight. They married, moved to Sebeka, and with the help of my prosperous, thrifty grandfather, opened a restaurant. They eventually raised five children and some of us were put to work.

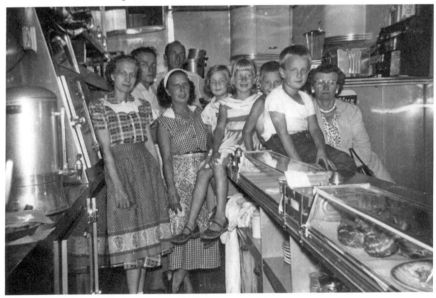

My job was filling the pop cooler. (I was small enough to reach easily into the lower cooler.) For my labor, I earned a nickel and a pick from the well stocked cooler. When RC Cola made the big jump to 16 ounces, it replaced my usual favorite, Dr. Pepper.

Throughout the '50s, breakfast was a busy time at Jim's Cafe, particularly in the summer when tourists were traveling to the lakes in northern Minnesota (U.S. 71 goes from International Falls on the Canadian border to New Orleans.) My father did all the cooking and made everything from scratch. Eggs, potatoes, and chicken were fried in lard.

But the war and aftermath of war brought changes. My grandfather quit farming in 1949, the year milk had to be pasteurized. His only son, heir apparent to the farm, died of pneumonia during army basic training.

War had taken a big toll on America's highly skilled creamery workers. When rushed, inexperienced replacements produced tainted, deadly milk, "raw milk" was put on trial — not the dislocations of war.

Did the European warring of the 20th century — directly and indirectly — help kill off traditional farming, railroads, small town creameries, and healthy traditional foods like raw milk? It was German novelist Hermann Hesse who wrote:

> "The greatest threat to our world comes from those who want war, who prepare for it, and who, by holding out vague promises of a future peace or by instilling fear of foreign aggression, try to make us accomplices to their plan."

As the Great War brought great change, it diminished small towns like Sebeka. By 1959, both the freight and passenger trains had made their last trips through town, and the once prosperous Sebeka Cooperative Creamery — like those throughout small town Minnesota — faded out of business.

For my father, too, time was running out. A tireless worker, war veteran, and smoker, Jim was suffering with chronic angina — debilitating chest pain. Unlike my grandfather's "abundant table," my father grew up in Missouri during a time when food was hard to come by.

He decided to sell the busy restaurant and relocate to Minneapolis where he could continue his treatments at the VA. His doctor, a young intern from England, recommended a new experimental heart surgery. He warned my dad, "Without surgery, Jim, you could be dead in six months." Impatient to get on with things, my father opted for surgery.

September 23, 1959

My mother rose early on the day of surgery. The previous evening a neighbor had given her a copy of *Reader's Digest* with an article that was highly critical of this experimental surgery. A lot of veterans had already died on the table. Those who learned the truth were backing out and going home.

My mother rushed off to the hospital at 6:30 a.m., the first day of autumn, September 23, 1959. "If only I can reach the hospital in time," she said to herself. My mother didn't drive. The slow bus ride brought her to the hospital too late. My father had already been wheeled into surgery.

A kind lady from Iowa, whose husband was being treated for cancer, sat with my mother in the large, airy first floor lobby. They waited for hours. At 12:15 in the afternoon, my mother was finally called to the doctor's office. It was the worst moment of her life.

The lady from Iowa went with her, holding her up. The sincerely shaken doctor said he was very sorry; he had followed all procedures — he had tried everything — but Jim was dead. Hours of hand-to-heart resuscitation failed to revive his heart and stony arteries.

Surgery can be oversold to serve a failed hypothesis or to benefit a hospital or surgical team. Veterans like my dad were easy marks. Decades of smoking didn't help. But none of this mattered to my mother that day.

What she needed more than anything else was the kind, sturdy woman from Iowa — an Angel's presence — holding her up as she learned that her Jim and all hope were gone.

Ordinary people redeem with acts of love and powerful stories — if only we listen.

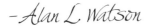

—Alan L. Watson

❧ *Notes* ❧

PART I: **The Test of Time**

1. "Hold the Eggs and Butter," *Time* Magazine, March 26, 1984.
2. David Phillips and Janet Moore, "For the heart of the boomers," *Minneapolis Star Tribune*, 12 September 2001, Sec. D, p.1.
3. Thomas J. Moore, *Heart Failure* (New York: Random House, 1989), p. 64.
4. Gary Taubes, "The Soft Science of Dietary Fat," *Science* Magazine, March 2001
5. Leila Abboud, "Expect a Food Fight as U.S. Revises Dietary Guidelines," *The Wall Street Journal*, 8 August 2003, Section B, p. 1
6. Ibid.
7. Ibid
8. Ibid.
9. Ibid.

Chapter 1: *Pyramid Schemes*

1. U.S. Department of Agriculture, *Home and Garden Bulletin* No. 1, Family Fare, Food management and Recipes, p. 3.
2. Ibid., p. 5.
3. Mary G. Enig, PhD, and Sally Fallon, "The Oiling of America." *Nexus Magazine*, Dec./Jan. 1999, Feb/Mar 1999. (Available at westonaprice.org)
4. Gary Taubes, *Good Calories, Bad Calories* (New York: Alfred A. Knopf, 2007), p. 32.
5. Ibid., p. 45-46.
6. Ibid., p. 45.
7. U.S. Department of Agriculture, Federal Nutrition Guidelines, Carbohydrates, Overview, p. 1.
8. Ibid., Fats, Overview, p. 1
9. Gordon M. Wardlaw, *Perspectives In Nutrition* (Boston: McGraw-Hill), p. 142

10. Russell l. Smith, Ph.D., *The Cholesterol Conspiracy* (St. Louis: Warren H. Green), p. 143.

11. Alice and Fred Ottoboni, "The Food Guide Pyramid: Will the Defects Be Corrected?" *Journal of American Physicians and Surgeons*, Winter 2004, Vol. 9, Number 4, p. 109.

12. Ibid., p. 110.

13. Gary Taubes, "What If It's All Been a Big Fat Lie?" *New York Times Magazine*, July 7, 2002.

14. Gary Taubes, "The Soft Science of Dietary Fat," *Science* Magazine, 30 March 2001: Vol. 291. no. 5513, p. 2539

15. *Good Calories, Bad Calories*, p. 72.

16. Ibid.

17. Gerald Reaven, *Syndrome X* (New York: Simon & Schuster), p.17.

Chapter 2: *Lessons of Framingham*

1. Thomas J. Moore, "The Cholesterol Myth," *The Atlantic Monthly*, September, 1989, p. 39.

2. Ibid, p. 40.

3. Ibid.

4. Ibid.

5. Uffe Ravnskov, MD, *The Cholesterol Myths* (Washington, DC: New Trends Publishing, 2000), p. 56.

6. Moore, p. 65.

7. Ibid.

8. Thomas Yannios, MD, *The Heart Disease Breakthrough* (New York: Wiley & Sons, 1999), p. 28.

9. Moore, p. 40

10. Bill Sardi, "The Cholesterol Conundrum." *Nutrition Science News*, September 1998, pp. 492-493.

11. John Carey, "Do Cholesterol Drugs Do Any Good," *Business Week*, January 28, 2008, p. 52-55.

12. Ibid.

13. Ibid.

14. Moore, op. cit., p. 65

Chapter 3: *Unintended Consequences*

1. Gary Taubes, *Good Calories, Bad Calories*, p. xviii
2. Ibid.
3. op. cit, p. xvii.
4. Andrew Weil, MD, *Healthy Aging* (NewYork: Alfred A. Knopf, 2005), p. 71.
5. Ibid., p. 70.
6. Ibid., p. 68.
7. Ibid., p. 69
8. Ibid., p. 148-152.
9. Robert C. Atkins, MD, *Dr. Atkins Age-Defying Diet Revolution* (New York, St. Martin's Press, 2000), p. 60.
10. Ibid., p.52
11. Weil, *Healthy Aging*, p. 72.
12. Ibid.
13. Atkins' *Age-Defying Diet Revolution*, p. 60.

Chapter 4: *Cereal Killer*

1. Sally Fallon, "Dirty Secrets of the Food Processing Industry," presentation given at the annual conference of Consumer Health of Canada, March, 2002. (available online at westonaprice.org).
2. Ibid.
3. Ibid.
4. Carol Simontacchi, *The Crazy Makers* (New York: Putnam, 2000), p. 106-109.
5. Ibid.
6. www.ctv.ca/servlet/ArticleNews/story/CTVNews/20060901/sugary_cereals_kids_060
7. Ibid.
8. www.universityofcalifornia.edu/news/article/16592
9. Gerald Reaven, MD, *Syndrome X, The Silent Killer*, (New York: Simon & Schuster, 2000), p. 18
10. Sally Fallon, *Nourishing Traditions* (Washington, DC: New Trends, 1999), p. 452- 454.
11. Ibid.
12. Ibid.

Chapter 5: *Class of 2018*

1. Jennifer Corbett Dooren, "Health Advisors Call for Action To Battle Obesity in Children," *The Wall Street Journal*, 1 October 2004.
2. Mark P. Becker, "No laughing matter, the obesity epidemic," *Minneapolis Star Tribune*, 8 November, 2003, p. A21
3. Ibid.
4. Jennifer Corbett Dooren.
5. Thomas Lee, "General Mills defends cereal ads," *Minneapolis Star Tribune*, 28 January 2005, Section D, p.1
6. Ibid.
7. Ibid.
8. Donna Halvorsen, "Dealing with Asthma," *Minneapolis Star Tribune*, 22 July 2003, Section E, p. 1
9. Jennifer Levitz, "Asthma Treatment Faces Revision," *The Wall Street Journal*, 11 May 2006, Section D, p. 3
10. Christine Goreman, "Born Too Soon," *Time* Magazine, October 18, 2004, p. 73
11. Bette Hileman, "Premature Births Rise 23% in U.S. Since Early 1980s," *Chemical and Engineering News*, 26 November 2001.
12. Gary Taubes, *Good Calories, Bad Calories* (New York: Knopf, 2007), p. 454

Chapter 6: *Loose Lips Sink Ships*

1. Kilmer McCully, Md, *The Heart Revolution* (HarperCollins: New York, 1999), p. 9
2. Ibid, p. 10.
3. Michelle Stacey, "The Rise and fall of Kilmer McCully," *New York Times* Magazine, August 9, 1997, p. 28.
4. Ibid., p. 29.
5. Ibid.
6. Ibid.
7. Stephen L. DeFelice, MD, *The Carnitine Defense*, (Rodale Reach, 1999), p. 129.

8. Stacey, p. 29.

9. Ibid, p. 28.

10. Atkins, *Dr. Atkins Age-Defying Revolution*, p. 32.

11. Ibid., p 32.

12. Stacey, p. 29.

13. McCully, *The Heart Revolution*, p. 10.

14. Ibid., p. 23.

15. Ibid., p. 11

16. Yannios, *The Heart Disease Breakthrough*, p. 40.

17. Ibid., p. 41.

Chapter 7: *Atkins without Atkins*

1. U.S. Department of Agriculture, Federal Nutrition Guidelines, Weight Management.

2. Alice and Fred Ottoboni, PhD's, *The Modern Nutritional Diseases* (Vincente Books, 2002), pgs. 77-80.

3. Taubes, *Good Calories, Bad Calories*, p. 414.

4. Ottoboni, *The Modern Nutritional Diseases*, p. 115.

5. Robert C. Atkins, MD, *Dr. Atkins Diet Revolution* (New York: McCay Co., 1972), p. 4

6. Walter Willett, MD, *Eat, Drink, and be Healthy* (New York: Simon & Schuster, 2001), p. 57.

7. Ibid., p. 58.

8. Atkins, *Dr. Atkins Diet Revolution*, pgs, 23-24.

9. Ibid., p. 26

10. Robert Davis, "Weight-loss doctor dies at 72 from head injuries," *USA Today*, April 18, 2003, p. 2A

Chapter 8: *Cholesterol is not a Medical Criminal*

1. Michael I. Gurr, PhD, *Lipids in Nutrition and Health* (Bridgewater, England: The Oily Press, 1999) p. 17.

2. Mary G. Enig, PhD, Know *Your Fats: The Complete Primer for Understanding the Nutrition of Fats, Oils, and Cholesterol* (Silver Springs, MD: Bethesda Press, 2000), p. 56.

3. Michael I. Gurr, PhD, *Lipid Biochemistry* (Oxford, England: Blackwell Science, 5th Edition, 2002), pgs 228-229.

4. Ibid.

5. Atkins, Dr. Atkins Age-Defying Revolution, pgs 24-25.

6. Ibid., p. 26

7. Ibid.

Chapter 9: *Lipids for Smart People*

1. Online: http://food.yahoo.com/blog/beautyeats/6971/the-ultimate guide-to-good-and-bad-fats

2. Enig, *Know Your Fats*, p. 36.

3. Gurr, *Lipids In Nutrition and Health*, pgs 13.

4. Ibid., p. 18-19

5. Ibid., pgs 1-2

6. Bruce Fife, Well Being Journal, March/April 2006, p. 21.

7. Ibid., pgs. 21-22

8. Ibid.

9. C.M. Seppanen and A. Saari Csallany, Department of Food Science and Nutrition, University of Minnesota.

10. Ibid.

11. Ibid.

12. The John R. Lee, *Medical Letter*, May 2002, p. 4.

13. Online Wikipedia: http://en.wikipedia.org/wiki/Acrylamide

14. Online Science Daily: http://www.sciencedaily.com/releases/2007/01/070116131545.htm

15. Online Weston A. Price Foundation: http://westonaprice.org/knowyourfats/interesterification.html

16. Ibid.

Chapter 10: *Praise the Lard*

1. Fran McCullough, *The Good Fat Cookbook* (New York: Scribner, 2003), p. 136.

2. Corby Kummer, "High on the Hog," editorial, *NY Times*, August 12, 2005.

3. Linda Joyce Forristal, "Put Lard Back in Your Larder," Wise Traditions in Food, Farming and the Healing Arts, Weston A. Price Foundation, Fall 2002.

4. Online: http://zarela.com/news/lard.html

5. Christopher Hirst, "Chefs prize it. The French love it. The Poles are hogging it. And now Britain's running out of it," *The Independent*, 31 December, 2007.

6. Jan Kwasniewski, *Optimal Nutrition* (Warsaw, Poland: Wydawnictwo, 1999).

7. Monica Eng, "Praise The Lard," *Chicago Tribune*, June 9, 2004.

8. Ibid.

9. Ibid.

10. Krispin Sullivan, CN, "The Miracle of Vitamin D, Wise Traditions in Food, Farming and the Healing Arts, Weston A. Price Foundation, Fall 2000, p. 11.

11. Ibid, p. 13

12. Ibid, pgs 14-15

13. Jim Suhr, "Corn-syrup industry seeks to sweeten image," *Minneapolis Star Tribune*, 11 September 2008, Sec. D, p.5.

❧ *Appendix 1* ❧

Lipid Panel — Summary of coronary heart disease risk factors

Ask your doctor for a complete lipid evaluation. In order to get reliable numbers, you must fast 10-12 hours before blood is drawn (you can drink water). Unless you are under age 50, total cholesterol and LDL are not reliable predictors of heart disease and are not delineated here.

Risk Factor	Optimum	Risk	Serious Risk
C-reactive Protein	<1	>2	>3
Fasting Glucose	87	>100	>110
Fibrinogen	<235	>235	>350
Homocystine	<8	>8	>12
Lipoprotein(a)	<20	>25	30
HDL (men)	>60	<50	<40
HDL (women)	>70	<60	<50
Triglycerides (TG)	<100	>100	>150
TG/HDL ratio	1:1	2:1	4:1

Total Cholesterol: Normal range 180 mg/dl to 350 mg/dl

C-reactive protein (CRP) is produced by the liver in response to inflammation in the arteries. If monitored early enough, elevated CRP can be an early warning of a heart attack six or more years in advance.

Fasting glucose is a measurement of how well your body is managing glucose or blood sugar. Ideal fasting glucose is 87.1. The high normal range (100 to 109) represents increased risk of heart disease.

Fibrinogen is the protein molecule that traps red blood cells into a blood clot. Elevated fibrinogen means thicker blood. Thicker blood flows less easily through partially blocked arteries. Consistent elevated fibrinogen — over 350 — conveys a 250 percent increased risk of heart disease compared to people with levels below 235.

Homocysteine is normally rapidly cleared from the bloodstream. Elevated homocysteine is a result of deficiencies of folic acid and vitamins B-6 and B-12. Elevated homocysteine damages arteries and dramatically increases the risk of heart attack and stroke. Levels greater than 8 micomoles per deciliter signal increased risk of heart disease.

Lipoprotein(a) has been called the "heart attack cholesterol." Lipoprotein(a) is actually a sticky protein that attaches to LDL and accumulates rapidly at the site of arterial lesions or ruptured plaque. Readings of 30 or more indicate serious increased risk of heart disease, especially in the presence of elevated fibrinogen (>350).

HDL is made by the liver and acts as a cholesterol mop, scavenging loose cholesterol and transporting it back to the liver for recycling. HDL is associated with protection from heart attacks. You want as much HDL as possible. HDL of 60 or more protects men — 70 or more protects women.

Triglycerides — like fasting glucose — should be under 100 mg/dl. Triglycerides are made in the liver from excess carbohydrates. Readings above 100 signal increased risk of heart disease. Risk is linear—the higher the number, the greater the risk, especially for women. Readings above 150 for both men and women mean sticky blood and a much greater risk of a heart attack.

TG:HDL ratio — The ratio of Triglycerides to HDL is the most reliable predictor of heart disease risk. Calculate your TG/HDL ratio by dividing your triglycerides by your HDL.

TG = 80	HDL = 80	ratio = 1:1	low risk of heart disease
TG = 200	HDL = 50	ratio = 4:1	high risk of heart disease

LDL Particle Size. There are seven sub-fractions of LDL and three sub-fractions of HDL. Testing for these sub-fractions is important for patients who have "normal lipid values" but persistent symptoms of heart disease.

LDL is a particle that consists of cholesterol and varying amounts of triglycerides. Steering the LDL is a protein called *Apoprotein B*. Because each LDL particle has an Apoprotein B marker, the number of LDL particles can be counted in a laboratory test. The cholesterol level in routine tests — milligrams of cholesterol in a deciliter of blood -does not reveal the number or size of the cholesterol particles.

At the same cholesterol level — say 220 mg/dl — a person can have a different distribution of LDL particle count and particle size. LDL "B" particles, for example, are smaller, denser, and contain more triglycerides, which induce chemical changes that make the LDL more much more likely to oxidize and damage artery walls.

If your triglycerides are low (below 75), your LDL is most likely the larger subclass A. If your triglycerides are elevated (over 150), your LDL is most likely the small, dense subclass B. High triglycerides are a warning sign that you may have this more oxidized-prone LDL — regardless of the level of cholesterol in your blood.

A fairly high percentage of people with aggressive heart disease have total cholesterol under 200. They could more accurately assess their risk by carefully scrutinizing glucose and triglycerides levels and by testing specifically for LDL subclass B.

❧ *Appendix 2* ❧

LIPIDS — THE BIG PICTURE

Far from being an inert food substance, it can be argued that fats are the most important of all dietary constituents. Our choice of kitchen fats may determine – more than anything else - whether or not we succumb to the three leading causes of death: Heart disease, cancer, and stroke.

Until recently, fats and oils have been viewed primarily as energy sources – and something to avoid. We now know that fats or lipids are a major component of our cell structure. Fatty acids control or police the life-giving flux of chemicals that go in and out of cell and organelle membranes – 24 hours a day!

In the words of lipid biochemist Michael Gurr:

> "Lipids occur in all cell types and contribute to cellular structure, provide stored fuel, and participate in many biological processes — ranging from transcription of the genetic code to regulation of vital metabolic pathways and physiological responses."

Throughout the living world, lipids or fats are shared by plants, animals, and microorganisms. As we have learned, there are no animal fats distinct from vegetable fats. As an example, your body can't tell the difference between oleic acid in lard and oleic acid in olive oil — they are identical.

Fat and fatty acid mean the same thing – a chain of carbon atoms in varying lengths from 1 to 24 carbons. Carbons form into chains by sharing electrons. When one pair of electrons is shared, a single bond is formed. Single bonds are chemically stable; fats with single bonds are called saturated fats.

When two electrons are shared in the carbon chain, a double bond is formed. Double bonds are chemically unstable. Monounsaturated fats have one double bond and are relatively stable. Polyunsaturated fats have two or more double bonds and are chemically unstable.

Because a lot of the fatty foods we've been told not to eat — avocados, bacon, butter, chocolate, coconut, eggs, olive oil, and red meat — contain a lot of monounsaturated and saturated fats, they are good for us!

The good news — these natural fats:

✸ Don't make you fat.

✸ Are nutrient dense, slowing the effects of aging

✸ Improve mood and memory

✸ Fill you up — not out

✸ Jump start your metabolism

✸ And — taste good!

Naming of Fats

Lipid biochemists use shorthand naming fats. As an example, 18 carbon saturated stearic acid is 18:0. The number before the colon is the carbon number; the number after is the double bonds. Eighteen carbon (18C) monounsaturated oleic acid is 18:1.

Type of Fat	Acid	Found In	Name	Crbns	Dbl Bnds
Saturated	butyric	butter	4:0	4	0
	caproic	milk fat	6:0	6	0
	caprylic	widespread	8:0	8	0
	capric	widespread	10:0	10	0
	lauric	oconut	12:0	12	0
	myristic	widespread	14:0	14	0
	palmitic	palm, lard	16:0	16	0
	stearic	beef, chocolate	18:0	18	0
Monounsaturated	oleic	olives, lard	18:1	18	1
	palmitoleic	chicken, lard	16:1	16	1
Polyunsaturated	linoleic	corn, soybeans	18:2	18	2
	alpha linolenic	flax, walnuts	18:3	18	3
	EPA	cold-water fish	20:5	20	5
	DHA	cold-water fish	22:6	22	6

Lipid Glossary

A1c test (short for glycosylated hemoglobin HbA1c) measures average blood glucose levels over a one or two month period. The test reveals damage or glycation to the oxygen-carrying hemoglobin (a protein) carried in red blood cells. HbA1c test results are expressed as a percentage, with 4 to 6 % considered non-diabetic.

Alpha linolenic acid (ALA) is the parent omega 3 (n-3) polyunsaturated fat with 18 carbons and three double bonds (18:3). ALA is classified "essential" because omega 3 is required in our diets in very small amounts. ALA is found abundantly in flaxseed and in lesser amounts in walnuts and unrefined vegetable oils. ALA is the precursor to EPA (eicosapentaenoic acid) which, in turn, converts into DHA (docosahexaenoic acid). EPA is a precursor to a series of short-lived jack-in-the-box hormones called eicosanoids (or prostaglandins). (EPA and DHA are found in fatty fish.)

Antioxidants are substances or compounds that slow or prevent oxidation reactions in food or in the body, particularly lipids. Antioxidants like fat-soluble vitamin E are especially important in preventing the oxidation of polyunsaturated fats in cell membranes. An antioxidant is able to donate electrons to electron-seeking compounds. As an example, Alpha Lipoic Acid is a versatile water and fat soluble antioxidant sold as a nutritional supplement.

Arachidonic acid (AA) is a very long chain omega 6 (n-6) polyunsaturated fat with 20 carbons and four double bonds (20:4). AA is formed in a healthy body from linoleic acid, the parent omega 6. Arachidonic acid is the precursor to a series of "eicosanoid" hormones and is found "preformed" in small but important amounts in liver, egg yolk, and butter, especially from grass-fed animals. (Google "Chris Masterjohn" to learn why AA may be "the essential omega 6.")

Bilayer describes the protective structure of biological membranes. These fatty bilayers guard cell membranes in all organelles (departments) within membranes. Fatty bilayers provide true homeland security. Saturated fats make up 50 percent or more of membrane and organelle bilayers.

Bile acid is synthesized in the liver from cholesterol. Bile is stored in the gallbladder and is released into the small intestine when fat is consumed. Bile plays an important role in the emulsification and absorption of fats. Bile is the only way cholesterol is excreted from the body — protecting us a final time by coating and stabilizing slow-moving feces.

Borage seed oil (starflower oil) is used as a dietary supplement because it is a rich source of conditionally essential GLA — gamma linolenic acid (20-25 percent). Your body converts omega 6 linoleic acid to GLA, but the conversion is uncertain. GLA is the precursor to anti-inflammatory, hormone-like eicosanoids.

Butter is an ancient, complex food consumed around the world for thousands of years. Made from the cream of cows, butter in the U.S. is 80 percent fat and 20 percent water. Butter contains a wide range of short- and medium-chain fatty acids (15 percent), including antiviral lauric acid. Butter made from cows grazing on grass is a particularly good source of vitamin A. *(See Milk Fat and Butter Composition, page 89.)*

Butyric acid (4:0) is a short chain 4 carbon saturated fat found only in the milk fat and butter from ruminant (grass-eating) animals. Short-chain fats are saturated fats that contain fewer than 8 carbons

Canola oil — or Con-ola — is a genetically engineered low erucic acid rapeseed oil originally developed in Canada and has been marketed in the U.S. since the mid 1980s as a "healthy oil." According to lipid biochemist Dr. Mary Enig, canola oil should be avoided. Animal studies indicate canola is associated with fibrotic heart lesions, negative changes in blood platelets, and vitamin E deficiency.

Capric Acid (10:0) is a medium chain 10 carbon saturated fat. Capric is widespread as a minor component. It is most abundant in coconut and palm kernel oils (4 to 6 percent) and is found to a lesser extent in the milk fat and butter from ruminant animals.

Caproic acid (6:0) is a short chain 6 carbon saturated fat found most abundantly in milk and butter and in very small amounts (less than 1 percent) in coconut and palm kernel oil.

Caprylic acid (8:0) is a medium chain 8 carbon saturated fat. Caprylic is a very minor component of most animal and plant fats. It is found most abundantly in coconut and palm kernel oils and to a lesser extent in the milk fat and butter from ruminant animals.

Carbohydrates supply calories to the body and include grains, fruits, vegetables, nuts, legumes and other plant foods. While our biological need for carbohydrates is zero, we don't want to miss out on the antioxidants and fiber in good quality fruits and vegetables. If you want to eat whole grains, learn how to buy, prepare, and serve them. (Best bet: *Nourishing Traditions* cookbook by Sally Fallon, president of the Weston A. Price Foundation.)

Chicken fat has a long history of safe use. It was used early last century in the U.S. as a pastry fat. And, yes, you can eat the crispy, delicious skin! A look at the composition chart below shows you what you would be missing. Chicken fat is an especially good source of antimicrobial palmitoleic acid (6 to 7 percent). As canola oil replaced chicken fat in Israel, diabetes rates have soared.

Chicken Fat Composition			
Percent	**Type/Acid**	**Chain length**	**# double bonds**
<1	lauric	12	0 Sat
1	myristic	14	0
23	palmitic	16	0
6	stearic	18	0
<1	myristoleic	14	1 Mono
6-8	palmitoleic	16	1
42	oleic	18	1
19	linoleic	18	2 Poly
1	alpha linolenic	18	3

Composition from *Know Your Fats*, Mary G. Enig, Ph.D

Cholesterol is a sterol (high molecular weight alcohol) that occurs widely in animal tissues as a vital component. Cholesterol plays a key role in regulating membrane fluidity, in effect, waterproofing our cells. Cholesterol also functions as an antioxidant, and is the precursor to all steroid and sex hormones, bile acids, and vitamin D. The human body contains about 100 grams of cholesterol — as much as 25 percent is in the brain. As Dr. Enig has pointed out, you can't eat enough cholesterol everyday to satisfy the body's requirements.

Chylomicrons are the largest lipoprotein. Lipoproteins deliver cholesterol and fat in the blood stream. Chylomicrons are synthesized in the gut from dietary fat and are released into the bloodstream via the lymph. Chylomicrons are identified by their protein marker, apolipoprotein B48 (apoB48) and are usually cleared from the circulation in two or three hours.

Cis-configuration is found generally in natural unrefined unsaturated fatty acids where the hydrogens are on the same side of the double bond — compared to the trans-configuration where, after high temperature, high pressure processing, the hydrogens jump across from each other at the double bond.

Coconut oil is extracted from the fruit of the coconut palm. It is a highly saturated fat (90 percent) with good baking and cooking properties. Coconut oil is a particular rich source of antimicrobial 12 carbon lauric acid (47 percent). Antimicrobial fatty acids are used by the body to kill or disable pathogenic viruses, bacteria, and protozoa. Coconut oil comes mainly from Indonesia and the Philippines.

Coconut Oil Composition			
Percent	**Type/Acid**	**Chain length**	**# double bonds**
8	caprylic	8	0 Sat
7	capric	10	0
49	lauric	12	0
18	myristic	14	0
8	palmitic	16	0
2	stearic	18	0
6	oleic	18	1 Mono
2	linoleic	18	2 Poly

Composition from *Know Your Fats*, Mary G. Enig, Ph.D

Cod liver oil is obtained from salt water fish with large livers and is a valuable source of vitamins A and D and provides the "elongated" omega 3 fats EPA (eicosapentaenoic acid) and DHA (docosahexaenoic acid.) Fish tissue oils contain EPA/DHA but do not contain the fat soluble vitamins. Cod liver oil is the most abundant source of vitamin D and is especially important in northern climates during the winter months.

Conjugated linoleic acid (CLA) is an 18 carbon fatty acid with two double bonds (18:2) found in small amounts in ruminant animals. Grain-feeding dramatically reduces CLA in milk and meat. Research at the University of Wisconsin demonstrates that CLA has many beneficial effects, including inhibition of cancer development and promotion of muscle development at the expense of fat.

Docosahexaenoic acid (DHA) is a very long-chain omega 3 (n-3) polyunsaturated fat with 22 carbons and 6 double bonds (22:6). DHA is abundant in fish and is found in small amounts in liver, egg yolks and butter, especially from grass-fed animals. DHA is a building block of tissues in the brain and the eye. DHA is formed in the body by a series of conversions that begins with alpha linolenic acid (ALA), the parent omega 3, but "preformed" DHA is very important for pregnant women and very young children. (Google "Chris Masterjohn" to learn why he feels DHA is the essential omega 3.)

Double bond is the name given to the linkage between two carbons (**C = C**) in the fatty acid chain when the two carbons share two links with each other instead of one. Carbons chains or fatty acids with double bonds are called unsaturated fats. Carbon chains or fatty acids with singles bonds (**C – C**) are called saturated fats.

Eicosanoids are short-lived, "jack-in-the box" hormones formed in the body from the parent omega 6 and omega 3 family of fats. (Eicosanoids function quickly within cell membranes and disappear.) A healthy 1:1 balance of omega 6 and omega 3 is important because different series of eicosanoids regulate a wide range of body functions, including the inflammatory process, arterial tension, and blood clotting.

Eicosapentaenoic acid (EPA) is a very long chain omega 3 (n-3) polyunsaturated fat with 20 carbons and 5 double bonds (20:5). EPA is formed in a healthy body in a series of steps beginning with alpha linolenic acid (ALA), the parent omega 3. EPA is most abundant in cold water fish such as herring, mackerel, salmon, and sardines. EPA is the immediate precursor to DHA and a series of eicosanoid hormones.

Endothelium is the single layer of flat platelet-like cells that line the inner surfaces of blood and lymph vessels and the heart and come into direct contact with the bloodstream. The endothelial cells are vulnerable to injury from nutritional deficiencies, elevated blood sugar, and high insulin levels.

Essential fatty acids (EFA) are the omega 3 and omega 6 fatty acids classified "essential" because they must come from our diets. The basic omega 3 (n-3) is alpha linolenic acid and the basic omega 6 (n-6) is linoleic acid. Both the n-3 and n-6 fatty acids convert into families of very long-chain fats that in turn produce the eicosanoids. We need the essential polyunsaturated fats in small, balanced amounts from whole unprocessed foods — plant and animal.

Familial hypercholesterolemia is a rare inherited disorder found in approximately 5 percent of the population that results in extremely high elevations of total and LDL cholesterol.

Fasting glucose (blood sugar test) is a measurement of residual glucose traveling in the blood after a 10 to 12 hour fast. Optimum fasting blood sugar is 87.1. Fasting glucose over 100 is associated with increased risk of heart disease. Diabetes is diagnosed when your fasting blood sugar reaches 125.

Flaxseed is the highest source of alpha linolenic acid (ALA), the basic omega 3. Oil is extracted from the seed and is excellent as a salad oil but cannot be heated or used in cooking. Whole milled flax provides the oil plus: complex fiber, minerals, and the important anti-cancer plant lignans.

Free radical is a highly reactive chemical compound that has an unpaired electron that is created by radiation, toxins, processing of foods, and normal body metabolic functions.

Gamma linolenic acid (GLA) is an omega-6 polyunsaturated fat with 18 carbons and 3 double bonds (18:3). GLA is considered conditionally essential because its production in the body from linoleic acid is uncertain. Trans fatty acids in the diet and conditions such as high blood sugar levels can block the conversion of linoleic acid to GLA. GLA is found in borage, black current, and evening primrose oil.

Glucagon is the complimentary/opposing hormone to insulin. While glucagon tells cells to release fat from storage and burn fat for energy, insulin tells cells to burn glucose for energy and convert excess glucose or sugar to body-made-fat. Dietary protein and fat signal the release of glucagon; carbohydrates call for insulin.

Glucose is the body's primary energy fuel (blood sugar). In pre-diabetics and diabetics, excess circulating glucose is a significant independent risk factor for coronary heart disease. Glucose is present in the sap of plants, in fruits, in honey, and is a constituent of starch and cellulose.

Glycerol is a 3 carbon alcohol molecule. It is the backbone of triglycerides (3 fatty acids attached to glycerol) and phospholipids (two fatty acids and a phosphate group attached to glycerol.) It is widely distributed in all living organisms.

Glycogen is the major store of carbohydrate energy in animal tissues, especially in liver and muscle cells. When carbohydrate storage is full, excess carbohydrate is converted into body-made-fat.

Heart failure (congestive heart failure) is condition in which the heart's ability to pump blood is impaired. Fluid can build up in the ankles, legs, lungs, and other tissues (edema). The incidence of heart failure has more than doubled since cholesterol-lowering statin drugs were introduced in 1987. At the same time that statin drugs interfere with cholesterol production, they also reduce the body's production of Coenzyme Q-10, a nutrient needed in highest concentrations in the heart muscle.

HDL (high density lipoprotein) is the most abundant lipoprotein. HDL is made in the liver and has the task of transporting "loose cholesterol" back to the liver for recycling. Because it is associated with protection from heart disease, HDL is usually referred to as "good" cholesterol." HDL, however, is not cholesterol — it is the most numerous lipoprotein and it carries cholesterol back to the liver for recycling.

Inflammation is the defense reaction of tissue to injury, infection, or irritation by chemicals or physical agents. As an example, excess highly processed vegetable fats easily oxidize in our bodies provoking inflammation in cells and tissues throughout the body. Coronary heart disease is now considered an inflammatory disorder. CRP (C-reactive protein) is a test that can provide early warning by detecting inflammation in the arteries years before a heart attack. An eight-year study of nearly 22,000 women published in the November 2002 *New England Journal of Medicine* found that CRP foretold heart attacks and strokes better than levels of LDL. Lead study director Dr. Paul Ridker said, "It's high time to move beyond cholesterol."

Insulin is a protein hormone secreted by the pancreas that promotes the uptake of glucose by body cells, particularly in the liver and muscles. Insulin regulates blood sugar levels in the blood and functions as a fat storage hormone. The resistance of body cells to the action of insulin is the beginning stage of Type 2 diabetes.

Interesterification is the latest method of modifying vegetable oil in an effort to replace "bad" trans fats. Interesterification is a highly industrial process that unnaturally rearranges the fatty acids in order to provide the oil with a higher melting temperature, longer shelf life, and "improved" baking qualities. The resulting product may be *trans*-free, but it will still contain chemical residues, solvents, and many dangerous breakdown products full of free radicals..

Ketosis is short for benign dietary ketosis. Ketosis is a natural biological process that results when glucose as an energy source is not available from dietary carbohydrates and the body switches to fat-burning. Fatty acids are released into the bloodstream and are converted to ketones, which are used by muscles, the brain, and other organs. Excess ketones are excreted in urine.

Lard has been used for centuries across the globe. Lard is similar to beef and lamb tallow, but it contains more unsaturated fat. The amount of unsaturated fat depends on what the pigs are eating. Lard is unusual in that 70% of the saturated palmitic acid (16:0) is in the 2-position of a triglyceride. In human milk, palmitic acid is also presented on the 2-position of the triglyceride. This suggests that lard or pork fat is very compatible with human physiology. *(See lard composition, page 101.)*

Lauric acid is a 12 carbon medium chain saturated fat (12:0) found in coconut and palm kernel oil. Nearly half of the fat in coconut is lauric acid. Dr. Mary Enig says lauric acid gives human milk "its major antimicrobial properties." Lauric acid is used in infant formulas and is effective against herpes, flu, hepatitis C, and HIV.

LDL (low density lipoprotein) is the main carrier of cholesterol in the body. LDL is the metabolic residue of VLDL, a lipoprotein made in the liver to transport liver-made-fat (triglycerides) and cholesterol. Often referred to as "bad" cholesterol, LDL only transports cholesterol. It is neither bad nor is it cholesterol.

LDL (Pattern A) is a subfraction of the lipoprotein LDL. Pattern A is a large fluffy triglyceride-poor LDL particle that is least likely to oxidize and accumulate in blood vessel walls. LDL subclass A is associated with triglyceride levels below 100.

LDL (Pattern B) is a subfraction of LDL. Pattern B is a small dense triglyceride-rich particle that is easily oxidized and more likely to accumulate in blood vessel walls. LDL subclass B is associated with elevated triglycerides.

Lesion is an injury to the artery wall, causing inflammation and abnormal tissue. Many things cause lesions, including high blood sugar, high insulin, elevated homocysteine, and the consumption of rancid, highly processed vegetable fats.

Linoleic acid (LA) is the 18 carbon essential omega 6 polyunsaturated fat with two double bonds (18:2). LA is a precursor to a family of fats including gamma linolenic acid, arachidonic acid, and three series of eicosanoid hormones. LA is needed in our diets in small amounts. LA is found in unrefined safflower oil (78 percent), sunflower seed oil (68 percent), corn oil (57 percent), and soybean oil (53 percent).

Lipoproteins transport cholesterol and fat in the body. Gut-made chylomicrons deliver reassembled dietary fat sent out from the intestinal wall, while VLDL delivers liver-made fat and cholesterol. LDL is the metabolic residue of VLDL and is the main carrier of cholesterol to the body. Made separately in the liver, HDL is the cholesterol mop and recycler.

Medium Chain Triglycerides (MCT) is a lipid product containing both medium-chain caprylic acid (8:0) and capric acid (10:0), usually derived from coconut and palm kernel oils. These medium chain fats — like short chain fats — enter the portal vein in the intestines and head directly to the liver. These fats are readily digested and may help utilize stored body fat for energy.

Monounsaturated fatty acids are long chain unsaturated fats that contain one double bond. Oleic acid is the most common monounsaturate, found abundantly in olive oil and in lard and poultry fat. Monounsaturated fats are safe for moderate heat cooking.

Myristic acid is a 14 carbon saturated fat (14:0). (Some researchers consider myristic acid a medium chain fat; some consider it long chain.) Myristic occurs widely in most animal and plant fats. Nutmeg butter is 70 to 80 percent myristic acid.

Oleic acid is the most common monounsaturated fat (16:1) found in plants and animals. In fact, when adipose tissue is analyzed, oleic acid predominates in the human body. Oleic acid is also the dominant fat in olive oil (see below). In the world of unsaturated fats, oleic acid is omega 9 (n-9) — not essential because our bodies can synthesize oleic acid.

Olive oil has the longest history of any plant oil. The oil is extracted from the fruit of the olive tree. Olive oil is the best vegetable fat for two reasons. First, you can press out the oil without resorting to high pressure, high temperature processing; second, olive oil contains both stable monounsaturated oleic acid (70 percent) and stable saturated fat (16 percent). Because it contains the full array of antioxidants found in olive oil, extra virgin olive oil — made from the first pressing — is best.

Olive Oil Composition			
Percent	**Type/Acid**	**Chain length**	**# double bonds**
14	palmitic	16	0 Sat
2	stearic	18	0
1	palmitoleic	16	1 Mono
71	oleic	18	1
10	linoleic	18	2 Poly
<1	alpha linolenic	18	3

Composition from *Know Your Fats*, Mary G. Enig, Ph.D

Omega is a term used to designate unsaturated fatty acids. If you see the term n-3, it is referring to omega 3. Omega 6 is designated n-6. (Other omegas are n-7 and n-9. Omega 3 and 6 are the essential fatty acids. (*See essential fatty acids, page 131.*)

Palm oil is obtained from the fleshy mesocarp of the oil palm fruit. Palm oil has been used for centuries in Africa and Asia. As you can see from the chart on the next page, palm oil is 50 percent saturated and 50 percent unsaturated. Unrefined palm oil is rich in carotenoids, tocopherols, and tocotrienols. Palm oil is an excellent, healthy oil that was "petitioned" out of our food supply in the 1980s by the collusive activities of the American Soybean Association and the Center for Science in the Public Interest.

Palm Oil Composition

Percent	Type/Acid	Chain length	# double bonds
1	myristic	14	0 Sat
45	palmitic	16	0
5	stearic	18	0
2	palmitoleic	16	1 Mono
39	oleic	18	1
9	linoleic	18	2 Poly

Composition from *Know Your Fats*, Mary G. Enig, Ph.D

Palm kernel oil is extracted from the inner seed of the palm fruit and has a fatty composition similar to coconut fat. Palm oil is a tasty and stable fat excellent for the production of baked goods and prepared foods. After the commercially charged "Anti Saturated Fat Attack" in the 1980s, trans-laden partially hydrogenated soybean oil replaced the much tastier, healthier tropical saturates.

Palm Kernel Oil Composition

Percent	Type/Acid	Chain length	# double bonds
4	caprylic	8	0 Sat
4	capric	10	0
50	lauric	12	0
16	myristic	14	0
8	palmitic	16	0
2	stearic	18	0
14	oleic	18	1 Mono
2	linoleic	18	2 Poly

Composition from *Know Your Fats*, Mary G. Enig, Ph.D

Palmitic acid is a 16 carbon saturated fat (16:0). Palmitic is the most common saturated fat in animals, plants, and microorganisms. Palmitic acid represents 68 percent of human lung surfactant. Palm oil is highest in palmitic acid (45 percent), but butter, chicken fat, cocoa butter, lard, and tallow are 25 to 26 percent palmitic acid. (Human milk fat is 20 to 25 percent palmitic acid.)

Palmitoleic acid is a 16 carbon monounsaturated fat (16:1) that is widespread in animals, plants, and microorganisms. Macadamia nuts are highest at 23 percent followed by cod liver oil at 12 percent. Chicken fat and lard are good sources. Fry your chicken, potatoes, and liver in lard and eat the chicken skin if you want to take advantage of palmitoleic's antimicrobial properties.

Partially hydrogenated fat is highly processed vegetable fat that has been chemically altered to prolong shelf life and to improve cooking and baking characteristics. Though trans fat labeling has forced food manufacturers to remove it from their products, it has been the fat of mass destruction in margarine and vegetable shortening since Crisco was introduced in 1912. Keep in mind that the "trans-free" commercial replacements for trans fats are just as bad or worse. All highly processed vegetable fats should be strictly avoided.

Phospholipids are a major component of cell membranes. The phospholipids and cholesterol provide flexible structure to membranes. Phospholipids consist of two fatty acids and glycerol (plus a phosphate group) while triglycerides contain three fatty acids and glycerol. In the brain, as an example, a high percentage of the phospholipids are saturated and monounsaturated fat. Lecithin is an example of a phospholipid that is found in all cell membranes.

Polyunsaturated fatty acids are long chain unsaturated fats that contain two or more double bonds. (Long chain fatty acids are between 14 and 24 carbons and can be saturated, monounsaturated, or polyunsaturated.) The basic omega 3 (alpha linolenic acid) and omega 6 (linoleic acid) are 18 carbon polyunsaturates. Commercial polyunsaturated fats should not be used for cooking, frying or baking.

Stearic acid is the common 18 carbon saturated fat found in beef, butter, cocoa powder and many other foods (18:0). Maligned by the American Heart Association as "an artery-clogging saturated fat," stearic acid raises protective HDL cholesterol and, in turn, lowers elevated triglycerides (blood fat) made by the liver from excess carbohydrates.

Statin drugs are cholesterol-lowering drugs with brand names such as Lipitor, Mevacor, Pravachol, and Zocor. Statins were introduced in 1987, the same year the National Cholesterol Education Program was made public. Statins inhibit or block an enzyme in the liver that produces cholesterol and Coenzyme Q10. Statins are to medicine what trans fats are to food: best avoided.

Tallow is the rendered fat from ruminant animals including cattle, sheep, or lamb. Tallow is a stable, safe frying fat that does not become rancid. No free radicals are formed from normal usage. McDonald's restaurants originally used beef tallow for deep frying French fries until several organizations within the U.S. prompted — even forced — their switch to trans-fat-laden partially hydrogenated soybean oil.

Trans-fatty acid (TFA) are unsaturated fatty acid that have one or more double bonds in the trans-configuration. TFAs are formed in the production of hydrogenated or partially hydrogenated fats. Hard margarine and vegetable shortening were a major source of trans fatty acids in the American diet for several decades.

Triglycerides *(technically triacylglycerol)* is the universal, common form of naturally occurring fats, both in the circulating blood and in adipose tissue. A common triglyceride is the binding of three fatty acids to a glycerol molecule. In blood work or a lipid panel, triglyceride has a different meaning. TG or TAG is a measurement of blood fats produced in the liver. Elevated triglycerides are a predictive risk factor for heart disease.

Please Note: It is important to mention that the information about the omega 6 and omega 3 essential fatty acids may not be totally accurate. The scientific history of the EFA's and their metabolic conversion products (i.e., arachidonic acid and DHA) is very short. Until recently, their low concentrations in living tissues and complex structures made them difficult to study.

❧ *Index* ❧

A

Advanced glycosylation end products: 29

American Heart Association (AHA): 8, 9, 12-14, 17, 19, 25, 27-28, 31, 33, 47, 72, 82, 88, 91, 99, 138

Antioxidant: 64, 127, 129

Apolipoprotein (apoB48; apo B100): 79, 129, 141

Apolipoprotein B100

Asthma: 7, 45, 47

Atkins, Robert C.: 3, 33, 35, 64, 67, 69, 75

Atkins diet: 7, 19, 75

B

Bacon:

B-48 apolipoprotein:

B-100 apolipoprotein:

Beef:

Bilayer, fatty: 127

Bile: 78, 129

Blood sugar: 28-30, 32, 34, 37-39, 47-50, 62, 69-71, 82, 92, 94, 95, 105, 127, 131-134

C

Carbohydrates: 13, 17, 28-32, 38-29, 48-50, 67, 69-72, 75-76, 80, 82, 105, 128, 134

Center for Disease Control (CDC): 7, 43, 141

Center for Science in the Public Interest (CSPI): 8, 93, 136

Cerami, Anthony: 29-30

Cholesterol: 5, 8-9, 14-15, 18, 22-25, 31, 39, 64, 76-78, 83-84, 129, 139

Chylomicron: 141

Circulation: 45, 74, 79-80, 129

Collagen: 29

Corn oil: 12, 20, 135

Crisco shortening: 87, 138

D

Diabetes: 7, 15, 18, 27-29, 31-34, 38-39, 43-48, 62, 65, 71072, 75, 82, 92, 95, 102, 105, 129, 133

Dietary Goals for the United States: 13, 141

Docosahexaenoic acid (DHA): 130

Douglass, William Campbell, M.D.: 16, 73

E

Eggs: 11-12, 40-41, 47, 50, 55, 63-66, 71, 78-79, 96-97, 102, 105, 126

Enig, Dr. Mary : 78, 90, 95-96, 107-108, 128, 134, 137

Essential fatty acids: 16, 65, 136

Exercise: 14, 21-22, 38, 53, 68, 73-74

F

Fallon, Sally: 35, 39, 96, 107-108, 128

Fats, monounsaturated: 92, 104, 126

Fats, polyunsaturated: 28, 88, 93-94, 126-127, 131, 138

Fats, saturated: 12, 16, 85, 88-90, 94-95, 106, 126, 128, 131

Fatty acid: 89-91, 97, 101-102, 130-131, 137, 139

Fat soluble vitamins: 11, 39, 79, 103-104, 106, 130

Food Guide Pyramid: 15-16, 142

Free radicals: 30, 74, 93, 139

G

General Mills: 42, 44, 47-48, 142

Glucose: 29, 31-32, 48-50, 65, 72, 79-80, 95, 132-133

Glycemic Index (GI): 48-50

Gurr, Michael: 78, 125

H

Harvard University: 18, 59, 69

Heart disease: 8-9, 12-16, 18, 21-25, 30-33, 38, 40-41, 45, 48, 52, 60-62, 72-75, 80-84, 90, 97, 105, 108, 132-133, 139

Heart Institute: 8

High density lipoprotein (HDL): 18, 32, 73, 76, 79, 81-83, 90, 95, 101, 133-135, 138

High fructose corn syrup: 14, 46, 48, 70, 106-107

High glycemic carbohydrates: 50

Hormones: 55-56, 68-69, 78, 127, 129, 131, 135

I

Insulin: 18, 28, 30-32, 34, 37-39, 45, 48-50, 53, 70-71, 95, 104, 131, 133

Insulin resistance: 30-31, 34

Interesterification: 133, 142

J

Jacobson, Michael: 17

K

Ketosis: 69, 134

Keys, Dr. Ancel: 12-13, 15, 59

Kraft Foods: 42, 44, 48

L

Lauric acid: 108, 128, 130, 134

Lard: 8, 11, 40, 65, 86, 88-89, 92, 94, 98-104, 106-107, 125-126, 134-135, 137-183

Linoleic acid: 56, 90, 94, 96, 127, 130-132, 138

Lipase: 79

Lipid: 79, 81, 90, 97, 126-127

Liver: 12, 37, 63, 70, 78-83, 94, 102-103, 127, 130, 132-135, 138-139

Low density lipoprotein (LDL): 25, 29-30, 32, 76, 79-83, 91, 132-135

M

Macular degeneration: 58, 64, 92-93

Margarine: 12, 14, 30, 87, 93, 96, 107, 138-139

McGovern, George: 13

McCully, Kilmer, M.D.: 59-62, 65

Metabolic syndrome: 38-39

Minneapolis Star Tribune: 44, 142

Monounsaturated fat: *(see fats, monounsaturated)*

Moore, Thomas J.: 21, 25, 142

Mottern, Nick: 13, 142

N

National Cholesterol Education Program: 8-9, 14-15, 18, 24, 31, 64, 76, 139

National Institutes of Health: 14, 21, 45, 60

New York Times: 100

New York Times Magazine: 17

Nurses Health Study:

O

Obesity: 7, 10, 15, 17-18, 22, 27, 31, 33, 37-38, 42-48, 50, 53, 67-69, 71-72, 75, 82, 85, 92, 105

Oleic acid: 101, 135-136

Olive oil: 86, 97, 100-101, 107, 125-126, 135-136

Omega 3 fat: 16, 56, 96, 102, 104, 127, 130-132, 136, 138

Omega 6 fat: 16, 90, 96, 101, 127, 131, 135, 138

P

Palmitic acid: 101, 137, 143

Pennington, Alfred: 70-71

Polyunsaturated fat: *(see fats, polyunsaturated)*

Price, Weston A.: 3, 39-41, 97, 103, 108, 128

Protein: 11, 29, 36, 38-40, 47-48, 50, 55, 64, 67-69, 71, 73, 75, 78-80, 87, 99, 102, 106, 129, 133

R

Reaven, Dr. Gerald: 18, 39

Risk factors: 22, 38, 63, 81

S

Saturated fat: *(see fats, saturated)*

Seven Countries Study: 13

Simontacchi, Carol: 37, 52

Stamler, Dr. Jeremiah: 12

Statin drugs: 23-24, 82-83, 133

Stearic acid: 18, 90, 100-101, 125-126, 136, 138

Syndrome X: 18, 32, 39

T

Tallow: 70, 85, 92-94, 107, 134, 137, 139

Taubes, Gary: 9, 13, 16-19, 27-28, 44, 48, 53, 69, 74, 85

Trans fatty acids: 87, 132, 143

Triglycerides: 32, 34, 39, 50, 80-82, 90, 95, 101, 132, 134-135, 138, 139

U

U.S. Department of Agriculture (USDA): 11, 14

V

Vegetable oil: 92-96

W

Wall Street Journal: 10

Weil, Dr. Andrew: 28-31, 33, 53, 67

Weston A. Price Foundation: 97, 108, 128

Y

Yannios, Thomas, M.D.: 23

Low Carb on the Web

Low Carb – Natural Fat – Real Food – Nutrition – Education - Consultation

Cereal Killer **Book Sales**

www.amazon.com (Alan Watson's author pages and blog)
www.dietHeartPublishing.com (Diet Heart Book Store)
www.innerglow.com/au (Australian distributor)
www.ppnf.com (Price-Pottenger Nutrition Foundation)
www.radiantlifecatalog.com (Radiant Life Company.)
www.nutribooks.com (wholesale distributor to U.S. health stores)

Health & Nutrition Education & Advocacy

✔ www.cholesterol-and-health.com – This site is dedicated to uncovering the truth about America's most demonized nutrients – cholesterol and saturated fat.

✔ www.dietHeartPublishing.com – Publisher of *Cereal Killer*. Website contains video and content dedicated to restoring America's traditional whole food high fat diet.

✔ www.naturallyknockedup.com – A great website dedicated to increasing the odds of conception through natural living and nourishing foods. Extensive resources for feeding and caring for children!

✔ www.nmsociety.org – The Metabolism Society provides research, information, and education in the application of fundamental science to nutrition - particularly dedicated to the incorporation of biochemical metabolism to solving the problems of obesity, diabetes, and cardiovascular disease.

✔ www.ppnf.org – Price-Pottenger Nutrition Foundation is committed to protecting, preserving, and disseminating the research of Weston A. Price, DDS, and Francis M. Pottenger, Jr., MD – and restoring America's traditional whole food high fat diet.

✔ www.westonaprice.org – Weston A. Price Foundation is dedicated to restoring nutrient-dense foods to the human diet. Members receive Wise Traditions, a quarterly journal dedicated to wholesome natural food, farming, and the healing arts.

Nutritional supplements

✔ **www.radiantlifecatalog.com** – Radiant Life's nutritional products and health equipment are the result of extensive research – including the very highest quality cod liver and butter oil. Radiant Life's mission is to offer products and resources that promote optimal health and sustainable living. (toll free: 1-888-593-8333.)

✔ **www.cayennecompany.com** – Since 1989, Cayenne Co (formerly Heart Foods) has manufactured herbal circulation formulas featuring High Heat African Birdseye Cayenne plus Ginger, Garlic, Onion, Hawthorn, and Gotu Kola. (toll free: 1-800-229-3663.)

Real Food-Quality Meat

✔ **www.eatwild.com** – A nationwide resource for safe, healthy, natural and nutritious grass-fed beef, lamb, goats, bison, poultry, pork, dairy and other wild edibles.

✔ **www.grasslandbeef.com** – Founded by fifth-generation farmer John Wood, U.S. Wellness Meats provides the highest quality foods inspired by a simple mission: "Do what's good for our animals, good for our planet and good for you."

✔ **www.minnesotagrown.com** – Minnesota's farm to table "buy local" food headquarters.

✔ **www.npofoods.com** – Nature's Prime Organic is a Minnesota-based provider of certified organic grass fed meat and poultry - plus the highest quality seafood delivered to your home or office.

✔ **www.realmilk.com** – An excellent website resource and advocate for Real Milk: Raw, whole – full-fat – and from grass-fed cows (fed pasture, hay and silage).

Natural foods & diet consultation…
because no one diet works for everyone.

✔ **www.jennette-turner.com** – Jennette Turner is a natural foods educator who has been teaching people to eat well and improve their health for over ten years. She works with clients in Minnesota and nationally – featuring an online meal planning program.

Natural foods & diet consultation...

✔ **www.marylangfield.com** – Mary Langfield is a Certified Holistic
Health Coach guiding busy professionals in Minnesota and nationally with ways to create happy, healthy lives. Mary will introduce
you to delicious and healthy food options and teach you how to
decode your body's cravings, reduce stress, and gain energy and
vitality for a long and better life.

Low Carb Blogs – Podcasts - Information

Amy Dungan
www.healthylowcarbliving.com
www.examiner.com/x-659-St-Louis-LowCarb-Examiner
www.carbsmart.com/low-carb-reality-by-amy-dungan.html

Jimmy Moore
www.livinlavidalowcarb.com
www.thelivinlowcarbshow.com (Don't miss this podcast)

Dr. Howard Peiper
www.kissyourlifehello.com (Live internet radio)
www.voiceamerica.com

Chris Kresser: www.thehealthyskeptic.org
Dana Carpender: www.lowcarbohydrate.net/blog
Dr. John Briffa: www.drbriffa.com
Dr. Kurt G. Harris: www.paleonu.com
Dr. Mike Eades: www.proteinpower.com/drmike
Dr. William Davis: www.heartscanblog.blogspot.com
Fred Hahn: www.slowburnfitness.com
Jennifer Eloff: www.low-carb-news.blogspot.com
Mary Langfield: www.mulberrymary.blogspot.com
Tom Naughton: www.fathead-movie.com

Go to **www.livinlavidalowcarb.com** (links) for a comprehensive list
of low carb resources on the internet.

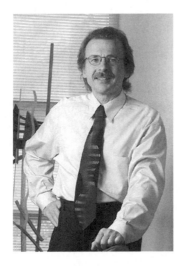

Alan Watson is a health researcher and a *Patient Advocate* with 20 years of experience in the nutritional supplement business. He is also the author of *21 Days to a Healthy Heart* (2002) — a groundbreaking book that includes an easy-to-follow 21 Day Plan to prevent and reverse diet-related heart disease.

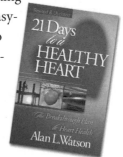

"*Cereal Killer* is well worth the read for those concerned with the health of a nation." — Midwest Book Review

"*Cereal Killer* is awesome! Thank you for the effort you put forth to promote a healthy lifestyle. You are doing a fine job!" — Jean Broeckx, Alberta, BC, Canada

"It is with great pride that we help promote this important and excellent book." — Joan Grinzi, RN, Executive Director, Price-Pottenger Nutrition Foundation

"...Watson brings a combination of food industry history, marketing and advertising, politics (oh, how important today), and large helpings of nutrition together in this very readable, interesting and potent book." — John Koenig, Writer, RXMuscle.com

"...Mr. Watson explains *diabesity*. I could barely put this book down. Mr. Watson's book is a great place to start and I highly recommend it." — Amy Dungan, Examiner.com

"We think this is a must read by anyone raising a family..." — US Wellness Meats Newsletter

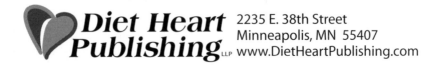

Diet Heart Publishing LLP

2235 E. 38th Street
Minneapolis, MN 55407
www.DietHeartPublishing.com